Inalva Valadares Freitas

Medicines Dispensing Practice:

Inalva Valadares Freitas

Medicines Dispensing Practice:

An Articulation of the Work Process in Family Health Programme Teams

ScienciaScripts

Imprint

Cover image: www.ingimage.com

This book is a translation from the original published under ISBN 978-3-330-99711-0.

Publisher:
Sciencia Scripts
is a trademark of
Dodo Books Indian Ocean Ltd. and OmniScriptum S.R.L publishing group

120 High Road, East Finchley, London, N2 9ED, United Kingdom
Str. Armeneasca 28/1, office 1, Chisinau MD-2012, Republic of Moldova, Europe
Managing Directors: Ieva Konstantinova, Victoria Ursu
info@omniscriptum.com

Printed at: see last page
ISBN: 978-620-8-61340-2

me

there's a time
rancid underneath
my verb

(Angelo Riccell Piovischini)

To the SUS users, people who never lose hope, and to the health workers who showed no resistance to sharing with us their experiences, hopes and despairs, their practices, their achievements and frustrations in the daily routine of health care, providing us with the opportunity to formulate this study as an instrument for reflecting on drug dispensing practices.

To the students of the Pharmacy course at UEFS who will soon take on the responsibility of transforming the current scenario of dispensing medicines into a humanised one, with the technique that guarantees the quality of care.

DEDICATORY

To my parents, my mother **Jacira Valadares Silva** who, with supreme wisdom and humility, taught me throughout my life the paths to follow and accepted with more teaching all the detours I took. To my father **Olegário Freitas Militão**, who for 39 years has accompanied me and looked after me from above.

To my daughter **Tâmara Combs,** who, even at a distance, followed my journey through the master's programme and gave me beautiful and wise examples of dedication and love for my studies.

To my sister **Ângela Valadares Freitas** (Pinha), an example of sisterly love and companionship, filling in for my absences and taking on my duties as her own.

To my brother **Ivonaldo Valadares Freitas** (Irmão), who always gave me a good laugh with his typical stories worthy of good, elaborate research.

ACKNOWLEDGEMENTS

To my family, my mum **Jacira,** my sister **Ângela,** my brother **Ivonaldo,** my daughter **Tâmara**, for their unconditional complicity in all the crazy things in my life, which have been many and continue to be many.

To Leozinho, **Leonardo Nascimento**, my grandson, for his material help in this work and who, without knowing it, gave me the exercise of tolerance and patience and at the same time was a victim of their absence.

To **Sonia Carine**, colleague, friend, special daughter, partner in joy and suffocation, and even more so in my diabrites.

To **Angelo Riccell Piovischini** for his constant joy, filling every moment of these two years with his joviality and also giving me the rediscovery and new joys of love and loving.

To my dear and special friends **Tatiane** and **Bruno,** yesterday my brilliant students, today my masters, who prepared me for this academic endeavour.

To Prof Dr **Maria Angela Nascimento** for all her teachings and example of professionalism and how it is possible to live with ideological and political differences in a respectful, harmonious and loving way.

Prof. **Tereza Coelho**, coordinator of the programme, for her lucid and sweet madness that gave me an immediate identity and an example to follow.

Professor **Maria de Nazareth Viana**, teacher, friend, responsible for my entry into academic life.

To my master's class, a unified example of a life project, responsibility, love of books, social commitment and the cultivation of friendship and joy.

My partners **Ionara, Carla, Lizziane** and **Dayene, who were** always close to me, lending me their youth and collegiality.

To **Neuza Chagas Araújo**, an employee of the Pharmacy Department, for her example of simplicity, coherence and loyalty.

To all my fellow lecturers on the Pharmacy course, for living together and learning what higher education is all about.

To my **dear students**, the main motivation behind my decision to study for a master's degree.

SUMMARY

Study on the Practice of Dispensing Medicines in Family Health Units in a municipality in Bahia. The objectives are to analyse the practice of dispensing medicines in the pharmacies of Family Health units in a municipality in the state of Bahia; to discuss the articulation of the Family Health team in the activities of dispensing medicines in Family Health units. Its theoretical framework is based on an understanding of the work process in public health. Qualitative research, from a critical analytical perspective, with 08 Family Health Units in a municipality in the state of Bahia, Brazil, as the field of study. The study participants were divided into three groups: Group I key informants (three); Group II workers (sixteen); Group III users (ten). The data collection techniques were systematic observation, semi-structured interviews and document analysis. Content analysis was used to analyse the data. The research was approved by the Research Ethics Committee of the State University of Feira de Santana, under opinion number 408.270. Observation and analysis of the data revealed a disjointed work process between the subjects, with a predominance of hard and soft-hard technologies, and a predominance of management activities to the detriment of user-centred care. The difficulties include the complete absence of pharmacists in the pharmacies of the Health Units, the inadequate structure of the pharmacies, and the lack of training of the agents responsible for dispensing, which makes it difficult to offer quality health care.

Keywords: Family Health Programme, Dispensing, Medicines, Health Care.

SUMMARY

CHAPTER 1 7

CHAPTER 2 13

CHAPTER 3 23

CHAPTER 4 35

CHAPTER 5 49

CHAPTER 1

INTRODUCTION

The social articulation of health work comes to mean, within the work process, the social needs to which it must respond (MENDES-GONÇALVES, 1992).

Our interest in studying the object of our research - the practice of dispensing medicines in Family Health Units, understood here as the practice of relations between men-individuals-workers with the objects and instruments of labour that should result in products, the reproduction of social relations in relation to the objects and instruments and the reproduction of the products, (MENDES-GONÇALVES, 1994), was motivated by 18 years of professional practice in a primary health care network in a municipality in the metropolitan region of Salvador.

This experience led us to reflect on the role of the professional pharmacist in the area of Collective Health, which contributed to some questions about our professional practice despite a health policy that did not see medication as a health good, but as a commodity handed over to drug entrepreneurs who promoted the proliferation of pharmacies throughout the country as a source of profit to the detriment of the population's health and care for the consequences of the abusive and trivialised use of medication.

The reality showed us that, on the one hand, in the basic network, we were concerned with meeting demands in the face of scarce resources, prioritising stock management, material resources and staff training, and, on the other hand, the search for a practice that was more directed towards the user of the medicine, valuing dispensing as a clinical act to be developed by the pharmacist, but without losing sight of the interrelationship between this professional and the individual and/or collective user.

However, these years of practice in the primary health care system motivated us to go beyond the normative managerial practice, characterised by the bureaucratisation of the service with involvement in drawing up consumption maps, distribution rules and so on, and to approach the health care team as a professional with the ability to contribute to an activity that is proper and necessary for users who, according to Barros (1995), are always exposed to the potential risks of the adverse effects of medicines and the consequences of their irrational and trivialised use, enriched by advertising and the excessive use of prescriptions after consulting a doctor.

Back then, in the 1980s, we were already active in trade organisations and in August 1988 we had the opportunity to take part in the First Meeting of Pharmaceutical Services and

Medicines Policy, which discussed topics such as drug research, drug industry patents, pharmaceutical industry patents, drug production, government regulation, the national list of essential medicines, among others (BRASIL, 1988). This was the first opportunity to discuss, albeit incipiently, the process and social division of labour in pharmacy, as the meeting was attended by various health professionals.

Despite the predominance of subjects relating to production, industrialisation, raw materials and others, the event gave hundreds of pharmacists and other participants the opportunity to ask questions about the current situation in the pharmaceutical sector, including demands for organised Pharmaceutical Services in line with the principles and guidelines of Brazil's recently approved Unified Health System (SUS).

At the end of the First Meeting on Pharmaceutical Services and Medicines Policy, the Letter from Brasilia was approved, in which we played a proactive role in the drafting of the document, noting the need to re-evaluate the concept of dispensing medicines, evoking its technical-scientific and social dimensions. The approval of this document (BRASIL, 1998) led to a plenary discussion with government technicians, researchers, university professors and students, parliamentarians and other segments present at the event, concluding with the approval of keeping the pharmacist active in all phases of the medicines cycle, with reinforcement for the dispensing stage, (highlighted by this researcher) as a technical-scientific activity of guidance on the use of medicines.

Changing the practice of dispensing, an activity defined in Law No. 5.991/73 as an "act of supplying the consumer with drugs, medicines, pharmaceutical inputs and related products, whether remunerated or not" (BRASIL, 1973), is becoming urgent, as it maintains a mechanical character, devoid of the pharmacist's involvement with the results to be achieved in pharmacotherapy. Based on this definition, dispensing is considered a legal activity that is exclusive to pharmacists, with Decree 85.878/81 in its entirety.

> Art. 1 - The following are the exclusive attributions of pharmaceutical professionals:
> I - dispensing or handling magisterial and pharmacopoeial formulas, when at the service of the general public or even of a private nature (BRASIL, 1981).

However, with some changes to the National Medicines Policy - PMN - (BRASIL, 1998), approved by Ministerial Order GM No. 3,916 of 30 October 1998, some advances in the definition of medicines dispensation are visible.

> The professional act of the pharmacist providing one or more medicines to a patient, usually in response to the presentation of a prescription drawn up by an authorised professional. In this context, the pharmacist informs and advises the patient on the appropriate use of the medicine. Important elements of guidance include emphasising compliance with the dosage, the influence of food, interaction with other medicines, recognising potential adverse reactions and the condition of the product.

With the institutionalisation of the Unified Health System, pharmacists played a leading role in the fight for a health policy that resulted in the approval of Law 8080 of 1990 (BRASIL, 1990), which sets out the conditions for the promotion, protection and recovery of health, the organisation and operation of the corresponding services and makes other provisions, including comprehensive therapeutic care, including pharmaceutical care, in Article 6(d).

At the same time as these movements and achievements, our practice in the Hospital Pharmacy area also contributed to our interest in research and the need to establish links between teaching and the practice of the profession that would gradually bring the management of medicines closer together, from their production to dispensing, as a clinical act focused on the benefit of the user, linked to health technologies, without losing sight of a user-centred practice.

Likewise, we observed that studies on the use of medicines show that there is a greater focus on administrative and economic aspects, the 'prohibitive' concepts of self-medication and the profile of users, evidenced in the studies *Rational* use of *medicines: an economic approach to decision-making* by Mota and others (2008), which details how pharmaceutical spending can be related to problems of scarcity, uncertainties in clinical decisions, and the preferences of prescribers; *Patients' knowledge of prescribed medicines after medical consultation and dispensing,* by Oenning, Oliveira and Blatt (2011), focuses on individuals' knowledge of their drug treatment without, however, addressing the clinical nature of dispensing.

Corroborating this line of study, Ramos, Silva and Alencar (2010) traced the quantitative and qualitative profile of medicines stored in homes in a municipality in the state of Bahia, without, however, mentioning the act of dispensing or the pharmacist's participation in this practice, which in our view reinforces the need for studies on the practice of dispensing, the final act in the medicine cycle.

When we left the exclusively technical activity of Pharmacy, we started teaching at the Pharmaceutical Sciences course at the State University of Feira de Santana-Bahia (UEFS) in 2001, having initially taken on the subjects of Social Pharmacy and Pharmaceutical Care , followed by coordinating the Knowledge Area and the Course Collegiate, unique experiences which motivated us to research and study the practice of dispensing medicines.

This motivation was also reinforced by the supervision of course completion work by undergraduate students in Pharmaceutical Sciences at UEFS focused on the study of the cycle of medicines, in general, taking as a reference the pharmaceutical assistance focused, for example, on studies by Gomes Junior (2009), which take an approach that is at odds with what we defend in pharmaceutical practice, given the prevalence of the use of medicines without a medical prescription, and the lack of coordination with public health policies, such as the Primary Care Policy, the Family Health Programme and the National Medicines Policy.

Added to these health care policies is the decision by the pharmaceutical profession's regulatory body to issue instruments that define the pharmacist's conduct with respect to the rights of users of medicines, guaranteeing services that lead to access and rational use of medicines based on the practice of dispensing medicines as the final act of health care. These rules are set out in Federal Pharmacy Council Resolutions 308, 357 and 542 (BRASIL, 1997; 2001; 2011).

However, the 'harmonisation' between legal norms and professional practice, particularly in the dispensing of medicines, is necessary, bearing in mind the Ministry of Health's spending on medicines for Primary Care programmes, which increased by 75% between 2006 and 2007, and on medicines for strategic programmes, which increased by 124% between 2002 and 2007 (VIEIRA; MENDES, 2009).

Therefore, given the complexity of this practice, we need to be attentive to the way in which health workers have been dispensing medicines, given that their work process has seen not only recent changes, but also the emergence of new work processes which, according to Merhy and Onocko (2006), are a consequence of technological incorporation into almost all professional practices.

In this context, Mendes-Gonçalves (1992) discusses, from a Marxist perspective, the social articulation of health work which, within the work process, comes to signify the social needs it must meet. As a consequence, we see the articulation between the different actors involved in the health work process, particularly in the practice of dispensing medicines, and the disarticulation between public health policies.

In addition, the reality leads us to reflect on the improvisation of activities and the understanding of the importance of active and pro-user dispensing, since there is no health teamwork, and the pharmacist often has numerous activities, including managing the unit, taking him away from clinical dispensing actions.

Given this scenario, we realise that this study on the practice of dispensing medicines in the pharmacies of family health units (USFs) in a municipality in the state of Bahia could contribute to the adoption of strategies and policies that improve the professional practice of pharmacists, as well as enabling the other people who work in dispensing to adopt a coherent and rational practice, which could consequently strengthen access to effective and safe medicines, as well as promoting their rational use with care directed at the individual and collective levels.

When we surveyed the data sources on studies dealing with the practice of dispensing, we saw that it has been little studied from the perspective of the clinical practice of using medicines. On the CAPES portal, in 2010, 2011 and 2013, we found no studies on dispensing medicines. When we accessed the LILACS database using the descriptors medicine and pharmaceutical care, we identified 70 studies ranging from a study of medicine prices to the incorporation pattern of antiretroviral training by the public health system in Brazil. As a result, when we used the word dispensation we found 120 articles and from these we cited those that, on initial observation, came close to our object of study.

The study by D'Ávila (2009) *on the dispensing of medicines in a Basic Health Unit in Belo Horizonte - MG*, concluded that there is no clinical practice of dispensing and, above all, with regard to the subjects of the study, it totally excludes the professional pharmacist.

In the same vein, Araújo and Freitas (2006), in their study *Concepções do profissional farmacêutico sobre a assistência farmacêutica na unidade básica de saúde: dificuldades e elementos para a mudança*, focus on the dispensing of medicines from the perspective of simple delivery and the administrative activities of pharmaceutical care.

The study *Atribuições do farmacêutico na atenção primária à saúde* (PHARMACIST*'s duties in primary health care)* (BARBOSA, 2009), treats dispensing tangentially as one of the pharmacist's activities and recognises that the presence of this professional at dispensing points is not necessarily linked to improvements in care for users, which differs sharply from the conception of our study, which establishes the presence of the pharmacist as the differential in the quality of care.

Thus, after surveying the different databases on the descriptors dispensing medicines, dispensing practice and dispensing, it became clear that when using the term dispensing, the most varied studies appear, from adherence to therapy (MENEZES, et al, 2012) to dispensing records as indicators of non-adherence, training of pharmacy technicians and analysis of prescriptions (MENEZES, et al; BEZZEGH; GOLDENBERG, 2011; GOMES; MACHADO; ACÚRCIO, 2009; VALADÃO; LISBOA; FERNANDES, 2004), which leads us to reaffirm our aim of emphasising the dispensing of medicines as a responsibility to be fully assumed by pharmacists in order to ensure the right to health.

Thus, as we have seen, there are few scientific publications on the practice of dispensing medicines. The study *Dispensing medicines from the specialised component in centres in Rio de Janeiro*, by Dellamora et al. (2012), concluded that the literature is poor in offering studies that discuss adherence to protocols and guidelines by pharmacists who could, through these, focus on the clinical aspect of dispensing practice.

Finally, we consider it relevant to study the practice of dispensing medicines as an important phase in the Pharmaceutical Services cycle. This practice is understood as a professional act by the pharmacist to provide one or more medicines in response to the presentation of a prescription drawn up by a legally authorised professional (BRASIL, 1998). With this in mind, we believe that this research can contribute to understanding dispensing as a clinical process that is also complex and involves practices, diverse knowledge and subjects from the perspective of the user's needs, in other words, a user-centred model.

We therefore came up with the following guiding **questions** for this study:

- How does the practice of dispensing medicines work in Family Health units in a municipality in Bahia?
- How does the activity(ies) of the Family Health team (doctor, nurse, dental surgeon) fit in with the medicines dispensing service?

In order to obtain answers to these questions, we have the **following objectives:**

- **To analyse** the practice of dispensing medicines in the pharmacies of Family Health units in a municipality in the state of Bahia;
- **To discuss** the articulation of the Family Health team in the activities of dispensing medicines in Family Health units.

CHAPTER 2

THEORETICAL FRAMEWORK

To build a model is to explore the contradiction, from mere denunciation to the verification of positive ways of overcoming it (MENDES-GONÇALVES, 1992, p.50).

In order to study the practice of dispensing medicines, we will analyse the phenomenon within the understanding of the work process as an activity inherent in all forms of social organisation, determined by the relations of the mode of production (MARX, 1994) which delimits the product as use-value, a material of nature adapted to human needs by changing its form.

To this end, we have recalled the Marxist theory that the human labour process differs from the metabolised activity of nature because this process already figures out its construction in the mind before transforming it into reality (MARX, 1994). Mendes-Gonçalves (1992) establishes a radical qualitative difference between the intentions of animals and those of humans, believing that the instruments of labour unequivocally attest to what is produced as a result of the labour process.

In this sense, when analysing the health work process, Mendes-Gonçalves (1992) identified that equipment, consumables, facilities and medicines are material instruments and also non-material instruments such as intellectual knowledge, which are effectively used in the work process and produce results that enter other work processes as objects of work, which will also constitute productive consumption.

However, Merhy and Onocko (2006) typify the different perspectives of health technologies by classifying them as hard, those characterised by machines and equipment; yeast, represented by structured knowledge; and light, those of interpersonal relationships, analysing the micro-politics of living labour.

In this respect, the health work process, in the study by Barros and Sá (2010), brings to light the weight of political, intersubjective and inconsistent micro-processes that point to a complexity conditioning the limits and possibilities of the production of care.

We therefore understand that dispensing medicines under the Marxist aspects and the analysis of Merhy and Onocko (2006) is an activity that involves the work process with the use of light and light-hard technologies, insofar as the transformation of work into a usable product makes use of material and non-material instruments, which are also complex because they involve various professionals, technologies, popular culture and organisational difficulties in primary care services as shown in the study by Alencar, Nascimento and Alencar (2011).

2.1 Pharmaceutical Care Practice

The study by Veloso (2010), Assistência Farmacêutica - discursos e práticas na capital do Império do Brasil, entre 1850 a 1880, aimed to discuss the health care provided by pharmacists during the 19th century in the city of Rio de Janeiro. The results reflect a practice characterised in that period that persists to this day, especially with regard to the restlessness of complementary practices that involved the art of formulating, preserving and selling, prescribing medicines and often applying therapeutic procedures that were common at the time.

In a broad concept of health, Barros (1995) quoted by Acurcio (2003) infers that the inefficiency of the Brazilian health system did not meet the real needs of citizens. Financial resources were mainly allocated to medical and hospital activities, with inputs, including medicines, being neglected, thus hindering the performance of the pharmaceutical professional.

Historically, Brazilian health policy has influenced the training of health professionals, including pharmacists, with a practice that distances them from the drug user, following the logic of the medicalising, biologist and hospital-centred model, centred on the drug, despite the fact that we consider the scientific knowledge needed to manage medicines to be important.

In the same way, this exclusive focus on the management of medicines is given not only in the training process for pharmacists, but also in professional practice, with Carvalho and others (2005) pointing out that these professionals have entered a phase characterised by an accumulation of theoretical knowledge about medicines without, however, translating into benefits for the individual and/or collective user, which reveals a practice centred on the 'product', far removed from the user who needs care oriented towards the use, risks and benefits of drug therapy.

During this purely theoretical phase, some questions were raised about the direction of the profession, its importance, social function, the training of professionals and the need to rescue the identity lost when the industrial boom turned medicine into a profitable product for commercial speculation.

The studies by Angonesi (2008) corroborate this statement, as they focus on the technical, legal and conceptual aspects of medicines, as well as questioning the practice in community pharmacies, those in the private sector and aimed at the general public.

The same is true of the legal definition of medicines, which has remained unchanged throughout time, meeting clinical, didactic and usual needs as technically elaborated pharmaceutical products for prophylactic, curative, palliative or diagnostic purposes (BRASIL, 1973), and is also, to this day, the main therapeutic resource used.

The impact of the use of medicines is not just biological; on the contrary, it ranges from the economic (market) to the health and social, and should therefore be considered from the perspective of a therapeutic tool and a consumer good (SEVALHO, 2003). However, as a consumer good, it is subject to trivialisation and pressure from advertising, the pharmaceutical industry and the mass media. However, according to Mota and others (2008), this trivialisation of the use of medicines as a symbol of health and a solution to all problems will require efforts to ensure that they are used rationally, i.e. appropriately for clinical needs, in the corresponding doses and at the lowest possible cost for everyone.

For Lyra Jr and Marques (2012), medicine has been perceived by society as a consumer good and a health promoter. It is therefore a product for sale on the market like so many other commodities, such as cars, televisions and so on, in other words, medicine consequently becomes or represents or symbolises that which produces health.

On the other hand, according to Araújo et al. (2005), the implementation of comprehensive pharmaceutical care, as advocated in Law No. 8.080/90, requires improvements that make it possible to assess its impact on the user's quality of life and the reduction of costs for the health system.

As a consequence of more advanced practices, Arraes, Barreto and Coelho (2007) have observed that in recent decades pharmaceutical practice has changed its focus. In view of this, these practices, which used to be centred on medication and are now more focused on the user of healthcare services, are characterised as being closer to the needs of the population and job market opportunities that increasingly require professionals specialised in the management of pharmacotherapy and therapeutic outcomes for the user, both individual and/or collective.

This is in line with the World Health Organisation (WHO, 1993), which in its Tokyo Declaration points out that the inappropriate use of medicines has consequences for both individuals and society in general. In this sense, pharmacists must be effective in meeting the essential needs of individuals and society.

In Brazil, with the advent of the Unified Health System (BRASIL, 1990) and the development of health policies such as the National Primary Care Policy - PNAB (BRASIL, 2006), the National Pharmaceutical Assistance Policy - PNM (BRASIL, 2004), society has a set of health actions at an individual and collective level and has achieved better conditions of access to medicines. In the same vein, Decree No. 7.508 of 28 July 2011 (BRASIL, 2011c), which provides for the organisation of the Unified Health System (SUS), health planning, health care and inter-federative coordination, and makes other provisions, expands access to specialised medicines, as set out in the Decree No. 7.508

of 28 July 2011 (BRASIL, 2011c), provides for the organisation of the Unified Health System (SUS), health planning, health care and inter-federative coordination, and makes other provisions.

> Art. 28. Universal and equal access to pharmaceutical care presupposes, cumulatively:
> I - the user is assisted by SUS health actions and services;
> II - the medicine has been prescribed by a health professional in the regular exercise of their duties in the SUS;
> III - the prescription complies with the RENAME and the Clinical Protocols and Therapeutic Guidelines or with the specific complementary state, district or municipal list of medicines; and
> IV - have the dispensation take place in units indicated by the SUS management.
> §Paragraph 1: The federal entities may expand user access to pharmaceutical assistance, provided that public health issues justify it.
> §Paragraph 2: The Ministry of Health may establish different rules for access to specialised medicines.

In order to develop the PNM, the executive branch used three basic guidelines: a) health regulation; b) economic regulation; c) and pharmaceutical assistance, the latter providing for the construction of therapeutic consensus on diseases and the indication of certain medicines (CARVALHO, 2010).

According to Araújo and others (2008), pharmaceutical care is an integral part of the primary health care system, in which the quality of the use of medicines is directly related to the quality of the health service, which is still related to the curative model centred on medical consultations and emergency care, with the pharmacy only meeting these demands.

In addition, other aspects are highlighted in the National Medicines Policy (BRASIL, 1998) which defines Pharmaceutical Assistance as:

> a group of activities related to medicines, designed to support the health actions demanded by a community. It involves the supply of medicines in each and every one of their constituent stages, conservation and quality control, the safety and therapeutic efficacy of medicines, the monitoring and evaluation of their use, and the acquisition and ongoing education of health professionals, patients and the community to ensure the rational use of medicines.

Pharmaceutical Services, defined in this way, involves several stages with the general aim of supporting health actions by promoting the population's access to medicines and their rational use and should be developed in a cycle that includes selection, programming, acquisition, storage, distribution and dispensing (BRASIL, 2004).

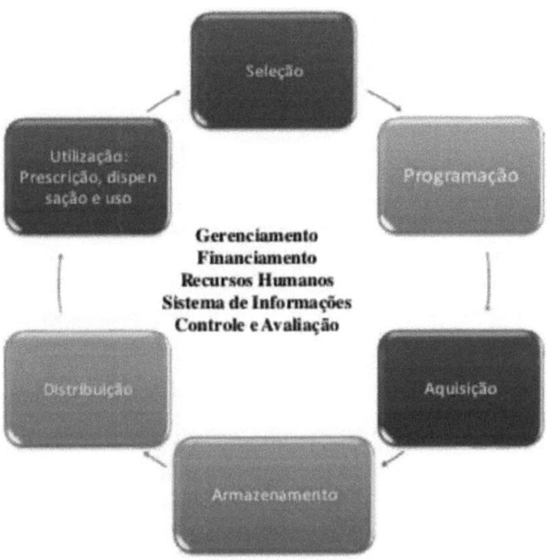

Pharmaceutical Services Cycle

The execution of each of these stages follows its own regulatory documents from the Ministry of Health and the National Health Surveillance Agency (ANVISA), such as a set of health standards, making the sector one of the most regulated, as shown by Nascimento (2005), and in the professional sphere, the resolutions of the Federal Pharmacy Council (CFF), which defines Pharmaceutical Assistance as

> [...] a set of actions and services aimed at ensuring comprehensive therapeutic care, health promotion and recovery, in public and private establishments that carry out design, research, handling, distribution, quality assurance and control, sanitary and epidemiological surveillance of medicines and pharmaceutical products (BRASIL, 1997, p.1).

In order to better study the dispensing stage defined in the CFF resolution, it is necessary to go through the other stages that precede it, since it is a cycle with interdependent and sequential stages.

The **production of medicines** can be considered the beginning of the medicine cycle and corresponds to obtaining pharmaceutical products from a set of knowledge and procedures conditioned to quality standards and techniques governed by regulations and norms (PERINI, 2003). Brazil has a network of official laboratories, a total of 21 belonging to the health secretariats of different states, the Armed Forces and foundations (MAGALHÃES et al, 2011), which make up the Brazilian Network of Health Analytical Laboratories - **REBLAS** (Brazil, 1999) and are associated with the Association of Official Pharmaceutical Laboratories of Brazil **(ALFOB)**, directing their production towards the basic health care network and specific programmes, especially the production of antiretroviral drugs.

This stage is followed by the **selection of medicines, which** is understood to be a fundamental activity, as it involves a process of choosing effective and safe medicines that are essential for meeting the needs of a given population (BRASIL, 2002). According to Alencar, Bastos, Alencar and Freitas (2011), selection makes it possible to create conditions for its adoption by maintaining an efficient and permanent process of objective and scientifically based information that guarantees the availability of medicines that meet the real demand of a community.

After selection, the cycle continues with the **medicines programming** stage, considered by the Ministry of Health (BRASIL, 2002) and Acúrcio (2003) as a set of activities designed to guarantee the availability of previously selected medicines to meet a certain demand for services in a defined period of time with a direct influence on the supply of and access to medicines.

On the other hand, Correr et al. (2011), in a narrative review on pharmaceutical care, believe that the medicine should be available at the right time, in optimum conditions for use and should be supplied together with information that enables the user to use it correctly.

Despite the stages of Pharmaceutical Services mentioned here, in this study we limited our research to the stage comprising DISPENSATION in live work in action, as defined by Merhy and Onocko (2006), meeting the needs within a quasi-structured process to achieve the objectives of educating about the correct use of medicines, contributing to the fulfilment of medical prescriptions and guaranteeing the supply of the right medicine in the right quantity (SOARES et al, 2013).

For Araújo and others (2008), the study Pharmaceutical Care in Primary Health Care addresses pharmaceutical care as a technological model in health that can be characterised according to the degree of technology, which converges with Mendes-Gonçalves' (1994) understanding that health technology is made up of knowledge and its material and non-material developments in the production of health services.

On the other hand, pharmaceutical care can be understood as being integrated into the process of health care and clinical management of medicines (CORRER; OTUKI; SOLER, 2011) and is related to health care and the therapeutic results effectively obtained, with the user of medicines as the main focus.

As a result, Alencar, Nascimento and Alencar (2011) agree that the construction of Brazilian health policies was marked by reflection on how to produce more resolutive actions, previously centred on controlling epidemics and focused on the disease and its cure, conforming to the biologising model. But they emphasise that the current context demands new forms of health care, considering that pharmacies have a responsibility as spaces for pharmacists' practices directly in the act of dispensing medication.

2.2 Medicines dispensing practice

The pharmaceutical care cycle has been studied by Marin (2003), Perini (2003) and Gomes (2012), mainly in the more administrative activities such as selection, administration, programming, acquisition, storage and distribution in compliance with the guidelines of GM Ordinance 3916/98 - National Medicines Policy (BRASIL, 1998), placing the clinical one, i.e. that centred on care for the individual, inherent in the practice of dispensing, second.

From the 1970s onwards, when the Central de Medicamentos (CEME) was created, it was responsible for promoting and organising the supply, at affordable prices or free of charge, of medicines to those who could not afford them at ordinary market prices, among other purposes. In the dispensing sector, care for medicines was directed exclusively at production and, as a result, regulations were restricted to raw materials, which were usually imported (BERMUDEZ, 1992). And beyond the public sphere, medicines were a matter for the market, with a lack of professional or sanitary rules and regulations.

Thus, the practice of dispensing medicines coexisted in a purely commercialised scenario, with medicine as a product for profit, the responsibility of industry, a mass producer of inputs and finished products (ROZENFELD, 2008), sidelining the practice of handling and dispensing medicines that were meaningful to the user. What's more, the search for new areas of professional activity, notably clinical analyses, came about in response to Brazil's private healthcare strategy and economic dependence, with a directive to acquire imported equipment for new pharmaceutical practices.

The study by Castro et al (2000) contributes to these new practices by focussing on some characteristics of the practice of self-medication, which requires greater attention from pharmacists, as does the study by Castro and Caldas (2011), which looks at the knowledge, practice and perception of the use of medicines.

However, in order to meet the evolving health care framework, particularly the new pharmaceutical practice, the Federal Pharmacy Council (BRASIL, 2001; 2011b) has issued resolutions that define and guide pharmacists to perform in accordance with the requirements of health policies and, more specifically, the practice of dispensing medicines, leading this professional to understand that dispensing is an active act of supplying medicines, for a fee or not, with the guarantee of rational use.

On the other hand, the dispensing of medicines in basic health networks has been done mechanically without due regard for the user's understanding of their health condition and their agreement with the treatment (ARRAES; BARRETO; COELHO, 2007). In this context, this situation refers to the perspectives and challenges of pharmaceutical care, defined as a component of the pharmacist's professional practice that requires direct interaction with the user in order to take care of their needs in relation to medicines (CIPOLLE; STRAND; MORLEY, 2006).

Through this practice, Angonesi and Rennó (2011) state that dispensing cannot be restricted to just delivering the medicine. The pharmacist must promote conditions so that the user uses the medicine in the best possible way and that this process ensures that all their actions are directed towards care.

Therefore, Soares et al. (2013) propose a dispensing model for the SUS that considers access as an attribute; reception, accountability, management and clinical pharmacy as the components for the rational use of medicines.

From this perspective, we corroborate Alencar, Bastos, Alencar and Freitas (2011) on the importance of re(signifying) the concepts of dispensing in order to bring about changes in values and attitudes within the pharmacy that reaffirm dispensing as an activity within the context of healthcare.

The study by Galatos et al. (2008) concludes that dispensing should be understood as part of the patient care process, i.e. as an activity carried out by a health professional with a focus on prevention and health promotion, with medication as an instrument of action.

In this way, the act of dispensing came to be recognised as part of the pharmacotherapeutic process, whether it be following a prescription or based on the user's decision. In this respect, the Política Nacional de Medicamentos (BRAZIL, 1998) provides a definition in which the commercial aspect of the activity is excluded, giving it a professional character that leads the pharmacist into a direct relationship with the user by understanding their needs and committing to the results of their pharmacotherapeutic design.

In order to do this, it is necessary to realise that the act of dispensing a medicine goes beyond the act of handing it over, because, in addition to offering some information, it must, according to Assis et al. (2010), involve relationships with users, thus building important moments that can produce contracts of accountability, reliability, bonding and welcoming.

Thus, we understand that dispensing practice must meet the needs of users based on the quality of the actions offered to them, clarifying doubts, encouraging adherence and the success of the prescribed treatment, because, according to Zanine and Oga (1994), medical prescription and guidance alone are not enough for users to use the medication correctly and understand the real need for it.

Consequently, Resolution 357 of the Federal Pharmacy Council (BRAZIL, 2001) requires the presence and performance of the pharmacist as an essential requirement for dispensing medicines to patients, whose attribution is non-delegable and cannot be exercised by mandate or representation as a way of guaranteeing that it will be provided with all the information necessary for the correct, safe and effective use of medicines according to the user's individual needs.

In the same vein, the advances made in the professional legislation of Resolution 542/2011 (BRASIL, 2011b) are manifested in the regulation of the dispensing of antimicrobials, with the pharmacist taking responsibility from Article 3 onwards for

> - The pharmacist's role is an essential requirement for dispensing antimicrobials to patients/users. This is a private activity and should include guidance on the correct use of these medicines.
> § Paragraph 1 - When dispensing any antimicrobial, the pharmacist must explain the benefits of the treatment to the patient/user in clear and detailed terms. They must also ensure that the patient/user has no doubts about aspects such as: I - reasons for the prescription, contraindications and precautions; II - dosage (dosage, dose, pharmaceutical form, technique, route and times of administration); III - mode of action; IV - adverse reactions and interactions;
> V - duration of treatment; VI - storage and disposal conditions.
> § Paragraph 2 - When dispensing any antimicrobial, pharmacists must consider that patient/user education/guidance is fundamental not only for adherence to treatment, but also for minimising the occurrence of bacterial resistance.
> § Paragraph 3 - In order to optimise dispensing, the pharmacist must be able to take action, develop communication skills and establish interpersonal relationships with the patient/user.
>
> § Paragraph 4 - The pharmacist must provide all the information necessary for the correct, safe and effective use of antimicrobials, according to the individual needs of the patient/user. (emphasis added by the researcher).

However, the evolution of standards is not accompanied by a practice committed to user care and, as a rule, is delegated to other professionals who are technicists and incipient in their clinical training (IVAMA et. al, 2001). Therefore, according to Cipolle; Strand and Morley, (2006) curricular reforms are needed to guide new practices in health care services, as well as following the new philosophy that guides the professional practice of pharmaceutical care in which the pharmacist is responsible for pharmacological therapy with the aim of achieving positive results that contribute to improving the user's quality of life.

It is therefore necessary to move forward with the Ministry of Health's proposal through the Secretariat of Science and Technology and Strategic Inputs (SCTIE), which has invested in training human resources with the aim of introducing the philosophy and practice of Pharmaceutical Care, which according to Cipolli et al (2006) is a component of the pharmacist's professional practice that requires direct interaction with the user in order to take care of their needs in relation to medicines.

Unlike the production of medicines, which makes use of hard technologies, dispensing is characterised by the use of soft technologies and as living work in action, as it requires the pharmacist to take responsibility for the user's needs and provide them with due care when dispensing, preventing and resolving Drug-Related Problems (DRPs), defined as any undesirable event presented by the citizen that involves or is suspected to have been caused by the medicine (CIPOLLE; STRAND; MORLEY, 2006).

Finally, these actions must meet the pharmacist's social practice in health care, requiring their inclusion in the health team as a professional in the field of collective health capable of contributing to the transformation of a humanised, resolutive and comprehensive health model.

CHAPTER 3

METHODOLOGY

Methodology requires reflection on the nature of the thing we want to know and an understanding of the problems involved in knowing it (CHAPELA; SERAPIONI; GASTALDO, 2012,p.587).

In this section we detail how the research was conducted, in other words, how we arrived at the results and understanding of how the practice of dispensing medicines in a family health unit is carried out, the deconstruction of our previous knowledge and understandings and how we went step by step putting together this new understanding of the reality being researched.

And in this sense, methodology is the instrument that helps us in the construction/reconstruction of knowledge, in the search for understanding, for a basis, for a foundation to understand, to interfere, to change, to reroute ourselves and our world (JESUS, 2010).

3.1 Types of Study

The study takes a qualitative, exploratory approach to the work process in the practice of dispensing medicines through a set of techniques and data processing. This process establishes a relationship between theoretical statements and objectified empirical data, not separating the subject who produces the knowledge from the object of study that will be constructed (ASSIS; JORGE, 2010). In this sense, qualitative research is a means of exploring and understanding the meaning that individuals or groups attribute to a social or human problem. In this respect, qualitative study is based on human relationships, opinions and interpretations, allowing social processes to be unveiled, new approaches to be built, new concepts and categories to be revised and created, and a direct identity between the subject and the research objective (MINAYO, 2010).

Consequently, Minayo (2010) warns against the use of specific and contextualised analyses, without the incursion of value judgements, but with the researcher establishing a critical view of their work. An exploratory study consists of describing a phenomenon in a given population, in a given period, providing a picture of how the data is related at that time, based on direct observation and information about the problem to which an answer is being sought, or discovering new phenomena or relationships between them (LAKATOS; MARCONI, 1996).

3.2 Context of the Study[1] : The municipality of Feira de Santana

3.2.1 History, Economics, Geography and Sociodemography

This research was carried out in the municipality of Feira de Santana, whose history can be

[1] Data taken from the IBGE (BRASIL, 2012).

traced back to the beginning of the 18th century, when the Portuguese Domingos Barbosa de Araújo and his wife, Ana Brandôa, owners of Fazenda Santana dos Olhos D'Água, had a chapel erected under the invocation of São Domingos e Santana. Around the chapel, the first tenant houses and slave quarters were built. On the death of the owners, these lands were later deemed vacant and incorporated into the National Treasury. Thanks to its geographical position, on the border between the recôncavo and the semi-arid tablelands and, therefore, at the confluence of the forest and coastal areas, the new settlement became a stopover for troops and travellers coming from the high hinterland of Bahia and the regions of Piauí and Goiás to the port of Nossa Senhora do Rosário de Cachoeira.

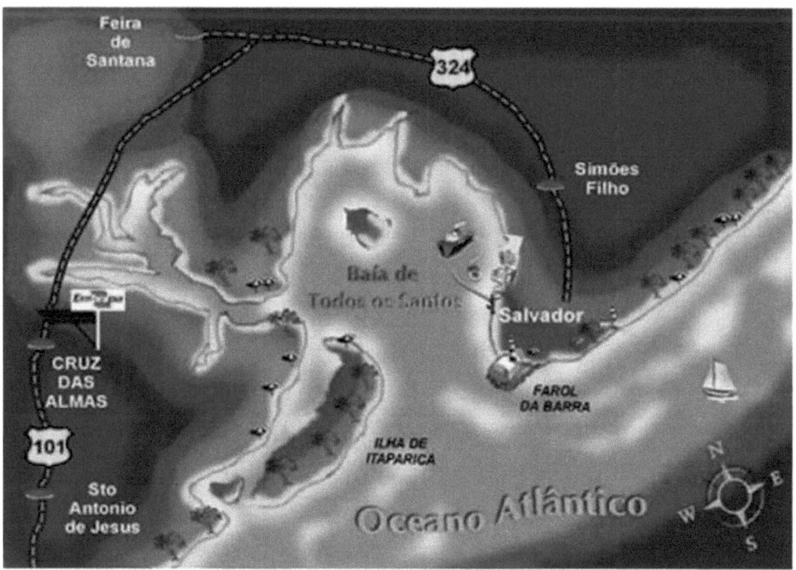

Figure 1 Map of the location of the city of Feira de Santana/Ba, 2014.
Source: Santos 2013 at http://www.klepsidra.net/klepsidra15/feira.htm

Even in the first half of the last century, the town began to become a centre for barter and trade. From there, the formation of the arraial - the arraial of Santana da Feira was a step. The incipient commerce gave rise to a small open-air fair held on the first

day of the week. The commerce that was established forced the opening of streets suitable for the traffic of market traders from all over. As a result, the population grew and shops sprang up. It was this impetus that led the inhabitants to request the creation of a municipality, which happened in 1832, with territory dismembered from that of Cachoeira.

The name Feira de Santana was determined by provincial law no. 1320 of 16-06-1873, which elevated the municipality to the status of a city and gave the seat the commercial name of Feira de Santana. The municipality played an important role in the federalist movement of 1832, rising up against the revolution that had broken out in the province of Bahia, and some of the Sabinada struggles took place on its territory. The great heroine of independence, Maria Quitéria, was born in the parish of São José das Itapororocas when it belonged to the municipality of Cachoeira. The locals[2] are called feirenses.

As of the territorial division dated 18-08-1988, the municipality is made up of eight districts: Feira de Santana, Bonfim da Feira, Governador Dr João Durval Carneiro, Humildes, Jaguara, Jaíba, Maria Quitéria and Tiquaruçu. This is how it remained in the territorial division dated 2005. According to the IBGE (2010), it has a population of 556,642 inhabitants in an area of 1,337.993 km^2.

Feira de Santana's poor population is concentrated in lower-class neighbourhoods and favelas such as Rocinha, Vietnã, Parque Lagoa do Subaé, Rua Nova, George Américo, Jussara, among others, and in expanding middle-class neighbourhoods and complexes such as Parque Tamandarí, Homero, Queimadinha and the famous Feira IX expansion.

In the socio-political context, around 17.3% of the population of Feira de Santana lives below the poverty line, a relatively low figure in the Northeast, while the capital, Salvador, has a poverty rate of 38%. Poverty in Feira de Santana, as in the whole of Brazil, mainly affects the less favoured classes such as blacks, migrants without professional qualifications and, reasonably, brown people (BRASIL, 2012).

Feira de Santana does not have large favelas or hillsides like most big cities. Most of the poor neighbourhoods and slums in Feira de Santana are in the

[2]Gentile: an adjective that designates an individual according to their place of birth or residence.

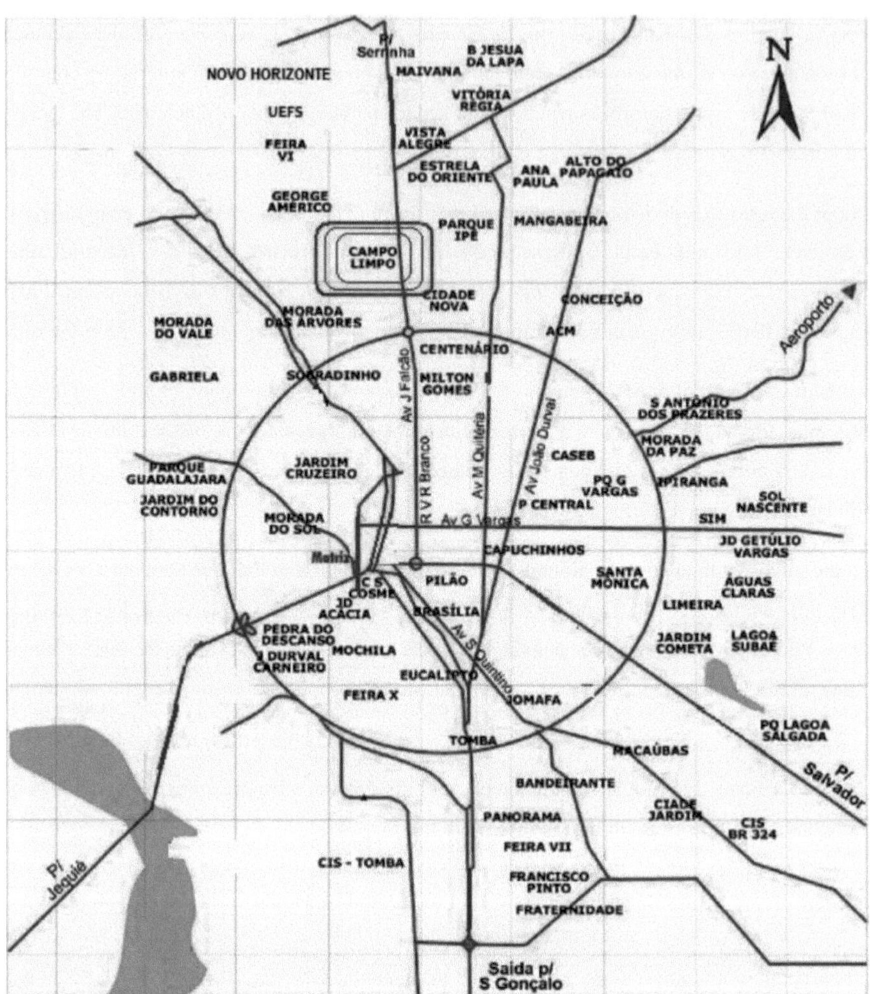

Figure 2 Map of the geographical distribution of the city's neighbourhoods
Source: www.google.com.br/ search? q=mapa+geografico+de+feira+de+santana&tbm=isch&source

The favelas have flat terrain and infrastructure such as paved streets, lighting, water and sewage systems, health centres and public transport - although a minority of the favelas in Feirense lack infrastructure. Figure 2 illustrates the geographical distribution of the city's neighbourhoods.

The municipality's health system is made up of 102 Health Centres/Family Health Units, 86 Family Health teams and 13 Health Centres; five Polyclinics and two Specialised Clinics, one Central Coordination of Pharmaceutical Assistance, eight Family Health Support Centre (NASF) teams, as part of the Primary Care Services Network. The population's coverage in relation to the Family Health team is 50 per cent. The municipality has been authorised to manage the Health System since March

2004, and this Management Commitment was reaffirmed in 2007 in the Management Pact (FEIRA DE SANTANA, 2013).

3.1.1 Field of Study Proper

The study itself was carried out in the Family Health Units (USF) of the municipality of Feira de Santana, since the dispensing of medicines is part of the comprehensive, therapeutic, including pharmaceutical care determined in Law No. 8.080/90, in line d of Article 6 (emphasis added by the researcher).

In order to select the USFs, we used some of the following inclusion criteria: - USFs with a full family health team; - USFs that have been in operation for more than six months; - USFs with a space exclusively for a pharmacy, located inside the health unit; - USFs located in both urban and rural areas; - USFs that are part of the Programme for Improving Access and Quality of Health Care (PMAQ), and with the monthly work of the Family Health Support Centre (NASF), making a total of eight USFs. Of the USFs selected, two operate in rural areas and six in urban areas. Only two have their own buildings and the others are rented. During the course of the research, we observed that all the units have territorial areas without community health agent coverage for different reasons such as: holidays, leave for health treatment and even resignation, without the proper replacement of staff by the Municipal Health Department (SMS).

The pharmacies in the USFs surveyed have inadequate structures for dispensing, characterised by their small size, lack of furniture for carrying out activities, and lack of qualified staff to carry out pharmaceutical care activities. All pharmacies are identified as such, even though the space is used for other activities. The therapeutic armoury available is varied, and all of them have medicines under special control (psychotropic drugs). The USF pharmacies do not have adequate temperature and aeration conditions, and there are spaces with apparent damp on the walls and direct sunlight on the medicines. We would also point out that in three (03) of them there are bars separating users from the attendants and dispensers of medicines.

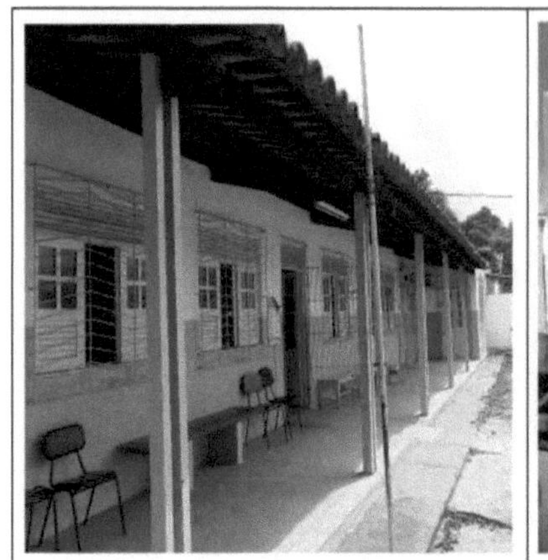
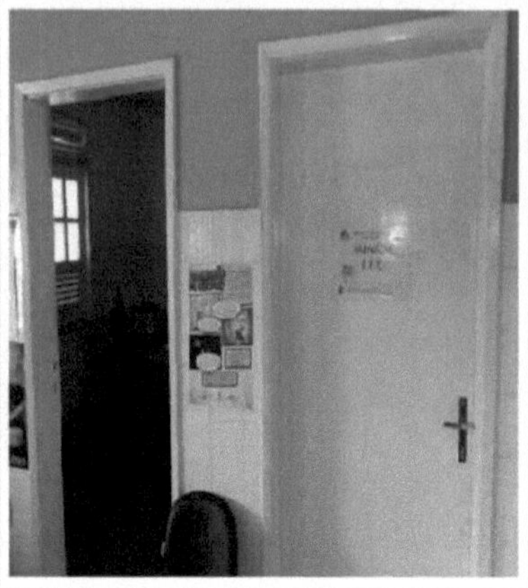
Facade of a Family Health Unit and identification of the pharmacy space.

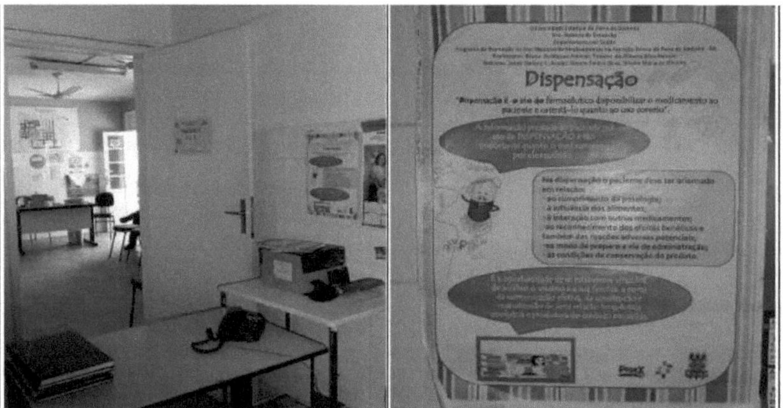

Interior of the pharmacy of a Family Health Unit and an educational poster on dispensing practices.

3.3 Study participants

The subjects taking part in the research are divided into three groups:

- Group I - key informants, made up of primary care managers represented by the USF managers, the Primary Care coordinator and the Municipal Pharmaceutical Assistance coordinator, totalling six key informants.
- Group II - health workers, regardless of their training, who work in the dispensing of medicines at the USFs selected in the study and other health workers who provide assistance and dispense medicines (doctors, nurses, dental surgeons, nursing technicians and/or assistants, pharmacists) who have been working at the USFs for more than six months, totalling nine workers.
- Group III - made up of ten users of the Family Health Units for more than a year over 18 years of age, for legal and ethical reasons, who seek the service to purchase medicines.

In order to arrive at a defined number of purposive sample subjects, the occurrence of theoretical saturation was taken into account. According to Fontanella et al. (2008), this happens when the interaction between the field of research and the researcher no longer provides elements capable of deepening theorisation and the researcher already has enough data to analyse the study and compose the results.

Therefore, according to Fontanella et al. (2008, p. 17), they say that,

> Sample closure due to theoretical saturation is operationally defined as suspending the inclusion of new participants when, in the researcher's judgement, the data obtained starts to show a certain redundancy or repetition and it is no longer considered relevant to continue collecting data. In other words, the information provided by the new research participants would add little to the material already obtained and would no longer contribute significantly to improving the theoretical reflection based on the data being collected.

Thus, the number of participants and USFs in this research were defined based on the occurrences of redundancy and convergence of meanings acquired during data collection. In total, there were 25 participants, represented in tables 1, 2 and 3 below.

Table 1 Profile of Group I - Key Informants (CI)

N°	Type of link with the SMS	Professional training	Total time working for SUS	Length of service in the Unit	Position held
1	Co-operative	Pharmacy	10 years	8 years	FA Coordinator
2	Co-operative	Nursing	10 years	1 and 2 months	AB Coordinator
3	Co-operative	Nursing	10 years	8 years	USF nurse
4	Co-operative	Nursing	12 years old	6 years	USF nurse
5	Co-operative	Nursing	12 years old	4 years	USF nurse
6	Co-operative	Medicine	15 years	8 years	Medical

Caption: AF:= Pharmaceutical Assistance; AB= Primary Care

Table 1 shows the composition of the key informants: one pharmacist, four nurses and one doctor. The managers' employment relationship is with the co-operative; their length of service in the SUS varies between 10 and 15 years. The length of service at the unit varies from one to eight years. The pharmacist and doctor occupy commissioned positions appointed politically by the city's mayor.

Table 2 Profile of Group II - Healthcare Workers (HCW)

N°	Type of link with the SMS	Professional training	Postgraduate studies	Total working time at SUS	Length of service at USF
7	Co-operative	Nursing	Specialising in Public Health	08 years	06 years
8	Co-operative	Nursing	Specialising in Public Health	More than 15 years	08 years

9	Co-operative	Nursing	Specialising in Public Health	12 years old	03 years
10	Co-operative	Nursing technician	No	06 years	02 years
11	Co-operative	Nursing technician	No	06 years	02 years
12	Co-operative	Nursing technician	No	06 years	02 years
13	Co-operative	Nursing technician	No	04 years	02 years
14	Co-operative	Dental Surgeon	No	04 years	02 years
15	Co-operative	Doctor	No	03 years	02 years

Chart 2 shows that of the workers who took part in this study, three are nurses, with more than three years' experience in the SUS and between two and eight years' experience in the USF. Of the nine participants, four are nursing technicians with two years' service in the USF and at least four years' experience in the SUS; one (01) is a dental surgeon and one is a doctor, both without postgraduate qualifications; all the nurses have specialised in Public Health and are employed through a cooperative.

Chart 3 Profile of Group III - Users (US)

N°	Sex	Age	Time spent at the USF	Level of education	Activity that exercises
17	F	36	More than 5 years	1st Grade	Housewife
18	F	42	More than 10 years	2° Grade	Trader
19	F	51	More than 8 years	2° Grade	Pensioner pen sioner INSS
19	M	40	6 years	1st grade incomplete	Trader
20	M	53	More than 6 years	1st grade incomplete	Ploughman
21	F	38	2 years	2° Grade	Housewife
22	F	26	2 years	2° Grade incomplete	Student
23	F	26	3 years	2° Grade	Housekeeper
24	F	31	4 years	1st Grade	Housewife
25	F	60	More than 10 years	1st Grade	Retired

Table 3 characterises the 10 users: eight are female, with an average age of 38; four of them have completed secondary school; three have completed primary school; two are traders; three are housewives; two are retired; one is a farmer; one is a domestic worker and one is a student.

The participants were identified by the letters of the category to which they belonged IC,T, U, followed by the number from 1 to 25, with the aim of respecting the anonymity of each one, in compliance with Resolution 196/1996 (BRASIL, 1996).

3.4 Data collection techniques

To meet the questions and objectives of this research, we used the following data collection techniques: systematic observation, semi-structured interviews and document analysis.

- Observation consists of following the work process of the subjects of this study in their work space. It is a technique for obtaining certain aspects of reality without the participation of the researcher, but it provides more direct contact with reality (LAKATOS; MARCONI, 1996).

The type of observation used was **systematic observation,** which according to Minayo (2000, p 134) "is one of the most widely used techniques in qualitative research" and followed a script that guided us through the aspects pertinent to the object of study. To this end, we drew up a script with topics directly linked to dispensing, such as observing the practice of dispensing medicines: the structure of the pharmacy in the family health unit; the initial reception and dialogue with the user; the organisation of the service; the storage of medicines; dispensing itself: the process of evaluating prescriptions; the use of soft technology; the use of soft-hard and hard technology (APPENDIX A).

The script, according to Lakatos and Marconi (1996), in addition to guiding the researcher, allows the answers to be compared with the same set of questions, making it possible to understand the point of view of the social actors envisaged as the subjects of the research.

We carried out 62 hours of observation in the eight (8) USFs that were selected in the months of August, September, October and November 2012. The content of these observations is included in item 4 Results and Discussions.

The second collection technique was the semi-structured interview, which allows the use of closed and open questions in which the interviewee has the opportunity to discuss the proposed topic without pre-fixed answers or conditions (SANTANA, 2010). To carry out the interviews, we also drew up three (3) scripts for each group of participants (Appendices B, C and D).

In order to carry out the interviews, we scheduled a time and place determined by the participants in a reserved space, free from listening and observation by other people

Confidentiality and secrecy were guaranteed during and after the interviews, which were recorded with the permission of the interviewee after signing the Informed Consent Form (ICF).

The third technique used was document analysis in order to enrich and complement the data from observations and interviews. According to Calado (2005), this involves consulting documents that should complement the object studied. We therefore used documents available at the USF, namely:

- Document 1 (doc. 1): Ministry of Health Ordinance No. 3,916 of 30 October 1998, which provides for the approval of the National Medicines Policy (BRASIL, 1998).
- Document 2 (doc. 2): Municipal Health Plan, 2010-2013;
- Document 3 (doc. 3): National Health Council Resolution No. 338 of 06 May 2004 approving the National Pharmaceutical Assistance Policy (BRASIL, 2004).
- Document 4 (doc. 4) A book recording the activities of the USF pharmacies, such as a list of medicines, requisitions for ordering medicines, stock control maps, a book recording the dispensing of medicines.

The documents analysed were included in the text according to the need to substantiate the observation or the data provided by the interviewees and are identified with their origin followed by the abbreviation (doc) and the number received.

1.5 Data analysis method

The data collected was analysed using the Content Analysis method, which is a detailed study of the words and phrases that make it up, looking for their meaning and intention in order to compare and evaluate them with the aim of clarifying the convergences and differences in the statements in order to extract their meaning (LAVILLE; DIONNE, 1999).

According to Bardin, quoted by Minayo (2010, p. 303), content analysis can be defined as

> A set of communication analysis techniques aimed at obtaining, through systematic and objective procedures for describing the content of messages, indicators (quantitative or not) that allow the inference of knowledge regarding the conditions of production/reception of these messages.

However, in Content Analysis we will follow the methodological path of Assis and Jorge (2010) based on Minayo (2004) from the three stages:

- Pre-analysis, the phase of organising the material, which involved recording and transcribing interviews, recording field notes, among other things, always reading in order to obtain guidance and impressions that emerged from the interviews, documents and observations.
- Analysing the material involved treating the material investigated through coding, classification and interpretation. This stage involves grouping and enumerating content, counting rules and defining categories (ASSIS; JORGE, 2010). To do this, we carried out an exhaustive reading of the data and then organised the horizontal and vertical summaries, identifying the differences in ideas. Based on this analysis, we constructed the empirical categories shown in tables 4, 5 and 6.

Table 4 Summary of Group 1 interviews - Key informants

NUCLEI OF MEANING	E.l	f-1	E.5	HORIZONTAL OVERVIEW
Understanding the practice of dispensation				
Work process in dispensing medicines at USFs -Agents -Objects -Technologies -Purposes -Management activities -Assistance activities				
Difficulties				
Facilities				
Progress				
Perspectives				
VERTICAL SYNTHESIS**				

* **Horizontal synthesis** refers to the interviewees' convergences and differences on each core meaning.
** **Vertical Synthesis** refers to each interviewee's general summary of the subject of the study.

Table 5 Summary of Group II interviews - Health workers

NUCLEI OF MEANING	E.l*	[...]	E.5	HORIZONTAL OVERVIEW*
Understanding the practice of dispensation				
Work process in dispensing disp ensing medicines in the USF -Agents -Objectives -Technologies -Purposes -Management activities -Care activities				
Difficulties				
Facilities				
Progress				
Perspectives				
VERTICAL SYNTHESIS**				

* **Horizontal synthesis** refers to the interviewees' convergences and differences on each core meaning.
** **Vertical Synthesis** refers to each interviewee's general summary of the subject of the study.

Table 6 Summary of Group III interviews - Users

NUCLEI OF MEANING	E.l	[-1	E.5	HORIZONTAL synthesis
Service you use at the USF				
Perception of dispensing practice -Agents -Objects -Technologies -Purposes -Management activities -Assistance activities				
Difficulties				
Facilities				
Progress				
Perspectives				
VERTICAL SYNTHESIS**				

* **Horizontal synthesis** refers to the interviewees' convergences and differences on each core meaning. ** **Vertical synthesis**

refers to each interviewee's general synthesis of the object of the study.

- The final analysis of the data allowed us to establish a link between the data collected and the theoretical frameworks of the research. To do this, we used triangulation of the data obtained from the interviews, observations and documents analysed, thus answering the questions that set out the research objectives.

Based on this triangulation of data and the comparison of the interviewees (Group I, Group II and Group III), we arrived at the following categories of analysis:

Category 1: SENSES AND MEANINGS OF DISPENSING MEDICINES IN THE PSF

Category 2: THE PRACTICE OF DISPENSING MEDICINES IN THE PSF: articulation of care and management activities.

1.6 Ethical aspects

As this is research involving human beings, we received a favourable opinion on the project and authorisation to carry out the research from the Ethics Committee of the State University of Feira de Santana. We would like to emphasise that we complied unreservedly with the ethical requirements set out in the Guidelines and Regulatory Norms for research involving human beings, contained in the Resolution of the National Health Council/MS 466/12 (BRASIL, 2012).

To this end, we drew up a Free and Informed Consent Form (FICF) which was always read and signed individually by the research participants (APPENDIX E).

The possible risks of this research were related to embarrassment, fear or feeling uncomfortable answering a question. Nothing was recorded until the end of the data collection.

The benefits of this research include the adoption of strategies and policies that help the pharmaceutical profession to promote better access to medicines and their correct use with better therapeutic results. In addition, the study should contribute to understanding dispensing as a complex clinical process that involves practices, diverse knowledge and subjects who aim to prioritise the user's needs.

The data collected will be used exclusively for scientific purposes, i.e. for dissemination and publication in scientific events such as seminars, congresses and periodicals in the form of articles, books and others.

CHAPTER 4

RESULTS AND DISCUSSIONS

Interpretation will never be the last word on the object studied, because the meaning of a message or a reality is always open in several directions (MINAYO, 2012, p.625).

When we studied the practice of dispensing medicines in family health units, we were aware of the complexity of the process and that, therefore, we would not be able to close the subject once we had completed the research, analysed the data and presented the results and discussions. We don't intend to arrive at a single truth, but rather to present elements that bring us closer to the reality of what happened with the participation of the study's subjects.

To this end, we have divided them into two analytical categories:

4.1 CATEGORY 1: MEANINGS AND SIGNIFICANCE OF MEDICINE DISPENSATION IN THE PSF: disarticulation between subjects and the work process.

4.2 CATEGORY 2: PRACTICES OF MEDICINE DISPENSATION IN THE PSF: dissent between theory and practice.

4.3 SENSES AND MEANINGS OF DISPENSING MEDICINES IN THE PSF

Based on the Marxist theory of labour, Mendes Gonçalves (1979;1992) applies it to the field of health. In the labour process, man's activity brings about a transformation in the object on which he acts by means of work instruments to produce products, and this transformation is subordinated to a certain end (MARX, 1994). Thus, the three component elements of the work process are: the activity suited to an end, i.e. the work itself, the object of work, i.e. the matter to which the work is applied, and the instruments or means of work, which constitute categories of analysis, therefore theoretical abstractions through which it is possible to approach and understand certain aspects of reality, in this study, health practices, whose work constitutes "the most fundamental basis for its realisation" (MENDES GONÇALVES, 1992).

From the perspective of this framework, understanding the work involved in dispensing medicines involves the theoretical basis, the inherent activities and those responsible, reflecting on the way in which the actions are carried out.

We can then see that the different understandings of dispensing medicines presented by the interviewees allow us to identify the objects of work (medicines and users) and from there another understanding that the pure and simple delivery of the medicine will guarantee the service and therapy to the users of the Family Health Units.

For the key informants that the dispensing of medicines

> [...] it's the act of giving the patient the medicine that has been prescribed with all the instructions. How to take it, if it's after meals, at night (IC,1).
>
> [...] it's having a good control of the stock of medicines so there's no shortage and no deviation, always talking and guiding the patient so they don't forget to use the medicine [...] this guarantees rational use, right? [...] (CI 4).
>
> [...] in order to have dispensation, we have to guarantee stock, control, correct ordering and talk a lot and provide **pharmaceutical assistance** [...] (IC3 3).

The key informants' understanding of dispensing medicines is close to the determinations of the National Medicines Policy (BRASIL, 1998 s/p, doc 1), which conceptualises dispensing as

> The pharmaceutical act of dispensing one or more medicines to a user, usually in response to the presentation of a prescription drawn up by an authorised professional. In this act, the pharmacist informs and guides the user on the appropriate use of the medicine. Important elements of this guidance include emphasising compliance with the dosage regime, the influence of food, interaction with other medicines, recognising potential adverse reactions and the product's storage conditions.

However, these statements do not reflect a complete and professional understanding of dispensing medicines, as they emphasise managerial activities, to the detriment of the user and the potential consequences of using medicines. However, the approximation with the concept of the PNM already points to a better understanding, considering that these are non-pharmaceutical health workers.

They are also unaware of the stages of the pharmaceutical care cycle, which includes dispensing medicines as an interdependent act of selection, programming, acquisition, storage and distribution, as a result of the reorientation of pharmaceutical care, for them a practice and not a public health policy.

For some health workers who take on activities and responsibilities that are not their own, according to these interviewees, dispensing takes on a mechanical dimension that needs to be done by someone else (TS 7). This situation reveals that both dispensing and pharmaceutical care are unknown to other health workers or are not even part of the content of other undergraduate health courses. This shows that even though pharmaceutical care is a set of multi-professional activities, it still doesn't take place in a way that is comprehensive and guarantees complete care and isn't just used as a technical term without a proper understanding of its impact on public health care.

Thus, for interviewee 3, a key informant, his actions are more collaborative and dependent on other professionals, and mainly reveal the impact of the absence of the pharmacist in the family health team, so that these same actions can be completed.

> [...] I take great care of the pharmacy and I count on the dedication of the nursing technician who is assigned to work only in the pharmacy, but I know that it would be much better if there was a pharmacist on the team and if he took care of the pharmacy. We feel the difference when the students are in the unit with Prof Bruno. We have more information, the nursing technician answers all our questions and the patients like to ask them lots of questions... (CI 3).

IC.3 conveys his concern about the complexity of the activity and the responsibilities he is taking on in this work process. The same is true of T.8, a dental surgeon, who is concerned about the use of medication and the implications of its use without dispensation by the professional directly and legally responsible for the act.

> [...] I'm always concerned about going to the pharmacy before prescribing the medicine, to find out if it's available in the unit, if the patient is going to take the medicine they need and I give them all the necessary instructions for correct use, but I know that the pharmacist should do this job, because they know a lot more about medicines than we do. I give instructions, but the patient may have forgotten everything by the time they leave the room, and the pharmacist is there at the end of the line and can give them the final instructions. Unfortunately, the government is the first to break the law. If a pharmacist is obligatory in private pharmacies, the public service should set an example and also have a professional on staff at all times when the unit is open[...]I have a lot of work, as do the nurses, so it's very important that every job is done by a professional with that knowledge. (T.8).

The statements made by IC.3 and TS.8 are in line with our observations of the difficulties pharmacy managers have in knowing which medicine is which when a different name appears on the packaging they have organised, for example, focusing on the importance of having a pharmacist present for dispensing.

The other health workers' view of dispensing medicines is mixed with an understanding of the division of labour and, at the same time, a mechanised conception of the act itself. Corroborating our observations, T.11, a doctor, states that:

> [...] I'm worried about whether the patient is using the medication correctly, I give them advice, but I can't get involved with the delivery of the medication. That's the nursing technician's job. I know it should be the pharmacist's job, but I don't get too involved with it... (T. 11).

Confronted with this information, the pharmacist from the municipality's pharmaceutical service revealed in an interview with the researcher that he intended to change this reality and make the manager aware of the need to hire more pharmacists and implement an organisation more focused on the data and actions that are developed to guarantee the availability of medicines in the network.

> [...] we need more pharmacists, there are so many activities before we get to dispensing... we do so many activities that don't appear to the other professionals and even less to the general public. For the patient, the doctor is everything, he doesn't even remember that we have to control the stock of the entire network, ensure that there is no shortage of medicines and that they don't expire on the shelves. Dispensing is being done, you just need medicines. We need pharmacists in the programme. You can't just think of the pharmacist when there's a shortage of medication or when it expires. We have to take care of much more. The logistics of purchasing, distribution and control (CI 2).

This statement is no different from the others, which have a reductionist view of dispensing, a mechanised and less important understanding, in that it does not demonstrate knowledge of the clinical act that involves dispensing medicines and which is expressed in the PNM as a

> The professional act of providing one or more medicines to a user, usually in response to the presentation of a prescription drawn up by an authorised professional. In this act, the pharmacist advises the user on the appropriate use of the medicine (BRASIL, 1998).

In this sense, prior to the PNM, the Federal Pharmacy Council, through the Resolution 308 of May 1997, which provides for pharmaceutical assistance, states in the

> Article 4 - It is the pharmacist's responsibility, when dispensing medicines, to interview users in order to obtain their medication profile; to maintain

> recording the pharmacotherapeutic records of its users, making it possible to monitor therapeutic responses; providing clear and comprehensive information on the correct way to administer medicines and warning of possible adverse reactions; providing information on the repercussions of diet and the simultaneous use of non-prescribed medicines; and providing guidance on the use of non-prescribed medicines (BRASIL 1997s/p).

In this sense, the statements converge towards a homogeneous view of dispensing as an exclusive act of the pharmacist, which is reduced to handing out the medicine and some guidance to users, as interviewees 7 and 9, nurses, report.

> [...] we take on various activities that don't belong to nurses, just out of respect for the user. We're not going to leave them without their medication, but that's the pharmacist's job. We already give guidance on the medication when it's administered here in the unit, but when they go home they need more guidance and it should be a pharmacist who does this [...] (T. 7).

> [...] I always advise the nursing technician in charge of the pharmacy to deliver the medicine with education and patient care, but she is not in a position to dispense it like a pharmacist who delivers the medicine and gives some guidance [...] (T. 9).

These statements are in line with our observations at the time of dispensing the medication, which was only delivered and accompanied by the instruction "take it as the doctor told you to". By understanding the dispensing of medication as a mechanical, merely bureaucratic act, they demonstrate the complexity of the act and the lack of coordination between workers in the health work process. Each has an understanding of their respective responsibilities and identifies with them, which are nursing care and medical care, without understanding what pharmaceutical care is and the important stage of dispensing medicines. However, by carrying out these activities, without knowing it, they are part of the pharmaceutical care work process and are important parts of this multi-professional process.

In this sense, articulation and integration must begin at the undergraduate level of the different health courses so that pharmaceutical care and all its stages and actions are understood as SUS care structures articulated with the other health policies and programmes offered by the state.

However, the absence of a pharmacist in the family health team contributes to this disarticulation and the existence of a gap both in care and in the health work process.

According to Mendes Gonçalves (1992), when studying the health work process, he emphasises that the elements of the object of the work, the instruments, the agents and the purpose of the work process must be examined together and not separately in order to configure a specific work process.

Interviewee 15's speech is surprising for its differentiated and broadened understanding and for bringing conceptual and assistance aspects regarding the dispensing of medicines and user-centred guidance.

> [...] the dispensing of medicines must be a clinical act in continuity with the medical act and articulated with nursing care, as a guarantee that the user is well cared for and that there will be satisfactory results from this care. The rational use of medicines will only be achieved when there is comprehensive care, with each of us knowing what the other is doing and complementing each other. [...]. I try to take part in all the meetings in the unit, listen to my colleagues and find out how and what each one does. We know that the department isn't worried about this at all, but if we don't do it this way, our work is worthless [...] (T. 15).

This statement leads us to another understanding of the pharmaceutical care actions that involve the pharmacotherapeutic profile, health education on medicines, home service with the use of medicines, pharmaceutical care, but which there is no record of being developed in the FH units, even in those that have pharmacists from the Family Health Support Centre (NASF). These actions are now part of pharmaceutical practice and should be integrated into SUS pharmaceutical care activities. Ivama (2002) explained in his proposal for a consensus that pharmaceutical care should be a model of practice developed in the context of Pharmaceutical Services, with a view to integrating health actions. Today, these actions are part of pharmaceutical practice and should be integrated into the pharmaceutical care activities of the SUS.

> [...] we can reach a very good level of pharmaceutical care. **Providing pharmaceutical care**, taking more care of the patient [...] without neglecting the selection part of

> purchasing, distribution... working more on health education, educating the patient about what medication is (IC.2).

The Federal Pharmacy Council (2011) also understands this and in Resolution No. 357 of 20 April 2011 regulates that

> Article 6, Subsection 6.22 Pharmaceutical Care is a concept of professional practice in which the patient is the main beneficiary of the pharmacist's actions. Care is the compendium of attitudes, behaviours, commitments, concerns, ethical values, functions, knowledge, responsibilities and skills in the provision of pharmacotherapy, with the aim of achieving defined therapeutic results in the patient's health and quality of life.
>
> Article 20 - the presence and performance of the pharmacist is an essential requirement for dispensing medicines to patients, whose attribution is non-delegable and cannot be exercised by mandate or representation.
>
> Art.31-The pharmacist must explain the benefits of the treatment clearly and in detail to the patient, making sure they are fully understood, adopting the following procedures:
>
> I- The pharmacist must provide all the information necessary for the correct, safe and effective use of medicines according to the user's individual needs.

In the light of the above quote, we can see the need for continuous improvement in drug dispensing practices in conjunction with other health care practices, in order to achieve a resolving action, making it possible to use everything available to eliminate suffering and the real causes of the user's problem (MERHY, 1994).

4.2 PRACTICES IN THE DISPENSATION OF MEDICINES IN THE PSF: dissent between theory and practice.

According to Mendes-Gonçalves (1992), the work dimension is the most fundamental basis for the realisation of social practices, although they are not reduced to this dimension. We therefore have a strong relationship between the conceptions of social practice and work. Dispensing medicines as a health practice involves work that is based on scientific knowledge, on one's own operative, technical or even technological knowledge (MENDES-GONÇALVES, 1994), but which requires reflection on its purpose and, therefore, its constituent elements, which must act in an articulated manner.

In our observations, we saw a disagreement between the practice observed and the interviewees' statements, which always refer to articulated teamwork, as seen in the statements by health workers when they say that they work as a team or emphasise the importance of teamwork.

> [...] here we work as a team, we always know what's going on in each sector. Everyone takes part in decisions and planning is done, from nursing needs for dressings to the scheduling of medicines [...] in special programmes everyone takes part (T.12).

> [...] the most important thing is to work as a team, everyone knowing everything, taking part in everything, knowing what each other is doing. On the day that one of us is absent, the patient won't suffer (T.14).

These statements are in stark contrast to our observations, including on a day of educational activities at the unit. At the same time as the nursing staff were giving a talk to nurses about contraceptive care, other workers entered the room, spoke loudly and called out to patients who were attending the talk, in a clear demonstration that workers confuse personal relationships with work relationships. The establishment of intimacy between them shows that there is no distinction between work and a formal activity. Instead of helping teamwork, this attitude hinders it. After the talks, we saw that everyone goes to their own space and carries out their activities without any connection to the other person's service, which reinforces the fact that there is no articulated or teamwork, insofar as there are no collective team interventions.

In this sense, we agree with Rocha and Almeida (2000) who draw attention to the need for an active stance of interrelation and interdisciplinary dialogue related to the various types of knowledge in a project to build care in solidarity. The validity of objective knowledge rests on the intersubjectivity experienced, on the success of establishing effective communication between the various subjects involved in these actions, in other words, on their expressive authenticity. We can see this divergence in the statements of the different agents, where there is only a hierarchisation of actions with centralised nursing supervision, as reported by interviewees 12 and 9.

> [...] I have peace of mind with the pharmacy, because the nursing technician takes very good care of it and if there's a problem she tells me. She's very strict with stock control, orders on time and every now and then I take a look at the books and everything is in order. She's the only one who looks after the medicines [...] (TS 12).

> [...] my job is just here in the pharmacy, looking after the cabinets of controlled medicines, checking the books every day. If anything goes wrong, I speak to the nurse and we sort it out, she tells me how to do it. [...] (TS 9).

Other statements try to establish the team character, but contradict our observation.

> [...] here everyone helps each other, on the day the medicines arrive, the colleagues come to help check and tidy up, but I'm the one who does the dispensing [...] there's work that everyone can't do because it's more of a mess than tidying up. I do everything myself, then I give the book to the nurse to keep track of. (TS 13).

During our observation we witnessed

> In one particular unit, the *nurses* (as they called themselves) were responsible for dispensing medicines, including access to the controlled drugs cupboard, and in order to ensure that there was no error in the use of medicines, I felt obliged to interfere in a dispensation, as there were three trainees dispensing and they were having serious difficulties identifying the prescribed medicine. This fact was omitted by the key informant when asked if pharmacy and nursing trainees were dispensing. In another unit, this happened again and I took the opportunity to observe and ask several questions about this practice, which did not differ from those carried out by the nursing technician,

> except for the concept that the *nurses* had about the legality and competences of dispensing medicines (Observation 1).

This situation is supported by the composition of the family health team recommended by the Ministry of Health (BRASIL, 2011c), which includes at least a general practitioner or specialist in family health or a family and community doctor, a general practitioner or specialist in family health nurse, a nursing assistant or technician and community health workers, with the possibility of adding oral health professionals to this composition as part of the multi-professional team: general dental surgeon or family health specialist, oral health assistant and/or technician, excluding from the minimum team the pharmacist and other workers important in comprehensive family care.

At another point in our observation, we saw that

> The Community Health Agents (CHAs) also freely access the pharmacy and take medicines out of the cabinets, then hand the prescription to the nursing technician, quoting names to be entered in the dispensation control books. It's a moment of unintelligible dialogue, with explanations and questions from one side to the other, even interfering with users waiting at the pharmacy door (Observation 2).

Key informant 6's account of what happened reveals that the CHWs do this type of activity to help patients who are unable to go to the USF and are assisted at home.

> [...] The CHAs know what each registrant uses and when they can't come to the unit, they are responsible for "picking up" the medication and bringing it to the next visit. But they can only pick up the medication if they have the prescription, which is transcribed. They're the ones in direct care and they know what the patients need [...] the pharmacy has to guarantee the medicine and keep track of it, especially for diabetic and hypertensive patients whose prescriptions are for continuous use (CI 6).

Observing these practices provides data on the disarticulation of health care and the work process, transforming dispensing into a mechanised act devoid of the humanisation needed in this care and neglecting guidance on the correct use of medicines, their implications and risks, precautions, interactions between medicines and the essential follow-up to record the effectiveness of the therapy.

Back in 1986, in our experience supervising pharmacies in the health network of a municipality in the metropolitan region of Salvador, during the Integrated Health Actions (AIS), we drew the attention of managers to the waste, low effectiveness and non-adherence to treatment as a result of dispensing medicines centred on managerial actions to register users in order to record productivity, to the detriment of the care needed when dispensing medicines. In reality, the absence of a pharmacist to meet the demands, including health education, due to the overload of administrative services, means that the actions of the CHAs have little effect on the correct use of medication and, possibly, insufficient results from pharmacotherapy.

Currently, the inclusion of pharmacists in primary care is significant, but their absence from the minimum FH team can lead to an overload of services for nursing staff, who are often not scientifically prepared to dispense medicines as a professional clinical act, capable of producing quality health care.

However, we would like to point out that these statements do not disqualify the dedication and work of nurses and nursing technicians, who are supported by Ordinance 2.488/2011 (BRASIL, 2011d), but this administrative delegation characterises a misuse of function, as it violates another legal provision, Decree 85.878/81 (BRASIL, 1981), which determines the dispensing of medicines as the pharmacist's private activity.

The disagreement between theory and practice encompasses other activities carried out within the scope of pharmaceutical care that are directly related to dispensing medicines, which are guaranteed in other legal provisions as exclusive and private activities of pharmacists, such as Law 5.991/1973, RDC No. 44/2009, which respectively provide for the trade in medicines, drugs, pharmaceutical inputs and correlates, and Good Pharmaceutical Practices. In addition, stock control, storage, dispensing and the issuing of documents to the health authorities are carried out irregularly or are not carried out at all due to the total lack of knowledge of the rules on the part of workers who are not performing their duties in the units.

Our analyses are corroborated by the following statements, which show the insufficient number of pharmacists in the network and the fact that there have been no competitive examinations to fill this need professional.

> [...] it would be important to have a pharmacist on the team, but the government is the first not to comply with the law. I know they do, but it's very little and they're not in all the units, we need this service, we can't do everything and there's a work overload as there isn't the right professional to do it. There are almost 120 units, all with a pharmacy and we don't even have pharmacists in 10 per cent of them... (IC.2).
>
> [...] A municipality of this size, a huge network and not having all the professionals is complicated and of course overloads the others. We also know that the law guarantees all the professionals, but we don't have them and we can't leave the patient without the medicine... [...] it's too much, but we can't talk about it openly because it's not our service (CI 4).

The reality once again reveals a regrettable situation and its consequences. There is no way of not spending a considerable amount of money on buying medicines and not getting positive results as the incorrect use of the medicine is repeated, with repeated returns to the units without the health problem being resolved, due to poorly orientated therapy and lack of the necessary care. The manifestations show interference in the work process without, however, establishing estrangement between the agents, but there remains a scenario of disregard and disrespect for the legal instruments that guarantee pharmacists the right to practice their profession and be part of the healthcare team. These provisions must be known to managers, who at the same time deny users the right to comprehensive and integrated care.

In the speeches of the group of workers, we identified with greater clarity the impact on the work process with the accumulation of activities and the absence of another professional, legally qualified to carry out the activities imposed on them in the process of job insecurity and low pay.

> [...] we want to do everything, to give the patient proper care, but it's not always possible because we have to do so much at the same time. What's more, we don't have stability, we can leave at any time, especially during elections when they cut everything, including staff. We need more professionals. You can't do healthcare with just doctors, we need pharmacists, nutritionists... (TS. 15).

> [...] we're everything here, I'm glad we get along, there's respect between us, but we know we're doing the job that should be done by someone else. We take good care of the patient, but it could be better if there were more professionals here. Everything is for nurses and nursing technicians (TS 14).

In this scenario and with such a compromised work process, the dispensing of medication does not follow the steps of evaluating the prescription in terms of its legal aspects; separating the medication and observing the expiry date; guidance on correct use; guidance on general care with the medication; recording care according to local rules and procedures that guarantee successful pharmacotherapy and concrete objectives for users, (ANGONESI; RENNÓ, 2012). The working conditions reported by health workers are also not conducive to good practice in all the stages of handling medicines, according to the following statements:

> [...] I'd like to do more for the user, but all the work here is manual, writing, there's no computer programme for stock control, patient registration. It takes time to check, count, record [...] (TS. 12).

> [...] I don't have time to talk to patients much. On the day the medicines arrive and also when the map is delivered, I can't pay much attention. I give basic instructions. (TS 15).

The words of these workers converge with our observations:

> While the user was waiting to be seen, the nursing technician carelessly took the prescription and continued talking to her colleague about the immunisation, how the vaccines were, whether the fridge was under control, which contradicts the information that she only looks after the pharmacy. The user stood waiting for ages and when he received the medicine, the professional didn't even look him in the face (Observation 3).

> In another unit we can see how much time workers spend on the hard technology of cutting material to recycle packaging, and they use creativity to make it easier to see the expiry date of medicines. All this intuitive work shows them the best way to store medicines and make it easier for them to dispense them (Observation 4).

Few times was it possible to observe and record attitudes that converged between doing and speaking. However, this does not disqualify the work of health workers, but it does reinforce the fact that precarious work interferes adversely with the quality and intentionality of dignified and humanised care.

On the other hand, the users' opinion of the medicines dispensing service apparently shows conformism, manifest revolt, as we can see in the statements of interviewees 17 and 21.

> [...] I've been a patient here for years, it's always like this, one day they have the medicine, another day they don't, another day they don't even look at us... it's not just their fault... there are too many people to attend to, right? Some people revolt because they have to buy the medicine, but I don't. [...] (U. 17).

> [...] I get angry with the government, we queue up and then they say they don't have the medicine, it's going to arrive, it's going to arrive and they don't even look at our house. I've lived here for over 30 years and I don't come to the health centre very often, because it's always like this. I try to use the poriclínica, where we take the medicine ourselves. You see this queue there, at this time of day, in the rain, and people don't say anything? Then when it breaks they think it's bad, I don't think so. Nobody wants to say anything (U. 21).

This situation becomes more complex and distant from users' needs when the medicine is part of the specialised component, requiring compliance with the Clinical Protocols and Therapeutic Guidelines (PCDT) for dispensing medicines, which often leads users to resort to the Judiciary.

> [...] the rigid dispensing standards adopted by the executive branch are pushing citizens further and further away from their constitutionally guaranteed right to health. The operation of the SUS shows that the state's supply of high-cost medicines has been increasingly restricted, controlled and curbed (CARVALHO, 2010 p. 165).

Our observations at this same USF reinforce what users have said:

> When I arrived at the unit before eight o'clock in the morning, there was already a queue, mostly women, the elderly, women with children and men on the sidelines. At eight o'clock, a worker from the unit arrived, already complaining about the queue. **For the dentist there's no ticket, you can get out of the queue. There are only Y forms for Dr X.** I noticed, because I'd been going to this unit for three days in a row, that this man was neither a technician nor a nursing assistant. He did a bit of everything in the unit. He was the only person in the unit at the time. I approached a few women and asked them to take part in the research. Of the more than twenty in the queue, none wanted to take part. They all said it was the first time they'd been to the unit, and they didn't know what to say, even though I explained the research, saying that their names wouldn't be disclosed. On that day, none of them took part in the survey. I despaired, because for me that was a rich moment to establish the contradiction. I digested my frustration and went on to devise another approach. I had already observed another moment of care without any humanisation, without an approach, shouting the person's name and complaining because the user didn't show up soon. It was a man with a wound, using a walking stick and with some difficulty getting around. He cursed, complained about the service and said that after waiting there for so many hours they wanted to hurry. At that moment I looked at a young man and approached him, successfully obtaining an interview and his consent to take part in the study. Here's what he said (Observation 5).

Below is an extract from the interview:

> [...] ôxe, it's always like this here, they treat us like animals, just because we're here in the countryside, far away from everything, but I say, don't treat me like that, I won't like it... I really say, this isn't theirs and this guy thinks he owns the post, he just talks like that. That's why I go to the clinics a lot, there's medicine there and they don't treat us like this. This is the end of the world." (U. 21).

For Lyra Junior and Mesquita (2012), this is when it is important to have a pharmacist with the competences and skills to turn dispensing into a practice of therapeutic relationships guided by ethical principles, mutual respect and, above all, co-responsibility from the perspective of comprehensive health actions.

In the same vein, Cordeiro and Leite (2008) emphasise the importance of the pharmacist's presence and the establishment of a communication channel between the pharmacist and other health workers for a multidisciplinary approach with the user as the total beneficiary.

The reasons that contribute to a model of care that lacks empathy and consideration for the user are justified by the workers as a result of working conditions, lack of space and equipment consistent with the service they offer, according to TS.10 and TS.16 below:

> [...] We do the pharmacist's job and we have nothing to help us. The nurse helps a lot and is always concerned about bringing information from the meetings at the SMS, but that's not enough. I have this book here so I can find the medicine and find out if it's the same one the doctor gave the patient. There's a book here that Bruno brought , but it's used by his students and can't stay in the pharmacy forever. You can't always go and ask the doctor what he's written. We don't have the internet to help us look for more information [...] it's paper, scissors and pen and that's it. When it's time to deliver the medicine, we have to count it, keep track of it, it's impossible, isn't it? (TS.10).
>
> [...] there should be a standardisation of the network and we should receive it and be able to inform the doctors, knowing how to deliver the medicine helps with orientation. But there isn't. Here in the unit we've already had some books that had everything about medicines and they've disappeared and no more have come. We do things according to what we learn in practice. Apart from the fact that we don't have any other conditions in which to work, the pharmacy is used for other services such as administering medicines, storing material that arrives from the secretariat, it's all cramped, with no space. (U.17).

This statement corroborates our observations of the use of soft-hard technologies, with a predominance of hard technology, the creation of their own tools to improve information and the work of stock control, control of the expiry date of medicines. Nailed to the wall of a pharmacy was a chart with a colour diagram for checking the expiry date. The tool was a little complex, but the lack of access to other sources of information encourages improvisation. In the units participating in the study, pharmacy workers only have one copy of the outdated Dictionary of Pharmaceutical Specialities (DEF), which is characterised by commercial information on medicines. The DEF is organised by the pharmaceutical industry and does not provide important information for dispensing and using medicines correctly.

The Ministry of Health publishes (BRASIL, 2002; 2004; 2006a; 2012b; doc. 3), through ordinances, various information instruments on medicines that help the work of pharmacists and all professionals who handle medicines and need to be up-to-date when dispensing medicines. Rename and the Therapeutic Formulary are regularly updated and standardised by ordinances or decrees, giving them credibility. There are also Clinical Protocols and Therapeutic Guidelines for the Specialised Component, both provided for in the National Medicines Policy. It is therefore up to the higher management to distribute these informative health policy instruments, which directly involve drug care, among all these units.

Observing this picture brings us to another situation, which is that public management does not excel in complying with public regulations. The medicines sector is considered to be the most regulated, with the aim of monitoring policies and guaranteeing the safety of medicines from production to final destination for the user. However, in the FH network, distribution and dispensing rules do not comply with minimum standards. Medicines under special control are free for any professional to access (doc.4), cupboards are often not locked, stock control and compliance with reports do not follow spreadsheets and control systems, nor do the professional regulations for pharmacists, such as the resolutions of the Federal Pharmacy Council No. 357/2001, which provides for Good Pharmacy Practices (BRASIL 2001); Resolution RDC No. 499/2008 on the provision of pharmaceutical services in pharmacies (BRAZIL, 2008) and, lastly, more recent resolutions such as CFF Resolution No. 586/2013 (BRAZIL, 2013), which regulates pharmaceutical prescription and other measures, and

Resolution No. 585, 2013, (BRASIL, 2013) which regulates the clinical attributions of pharmacists and makes other provisions. Logically, these instruments can only be complied with by pharmaceutical professionals, but when the public manager does not include this professional in the family health team, there is a compromise of all pharmaceutical care, the work process as well as relations in care and management activities.

Another aspect to consider is what kind of care is being offered to the SUS user population. From management to management, the picture repeats itself. According to Alencar (2013), previous studies

> conclude that managerial activities (selection, programming, acquisition, distribution, storage) predominate over care activities (dispensing and other pharmaceutical care activities, both of which are carried out without the necessary technical rigour, without evaluation and control by the PSF workers themselves, the Pharmaceutical Care Sector and other sectors of the Municipal Health Department (ALENCAR, 2013, p.161).

According to Araújo and others (2008a), the study on the profile of PS in primary care shows that solving the problem in general will not be simple if the way the service is structured is maintained. In specific terms, it is essential for managers to rationalise the use of medicines from prescription to use by the user.

In view of the above, the reality is that the work process is mechanised and lacks the pharmacist's competences and skills for dispensing, insofar as the pharmacist is not part of the minimum PSF team and even in the units that have the NASF team, the activities are disjointed and do not meet the needs of the non-pharmacist workers who take on the practice of dispensing medicines.

The difficulties in dispensing medicines mentioned by the workers predominate in the day-to-day running of the units and are listed as the lack of adequate structure in the pharmacies; the absence of a pharmacist on the team; the lack of equipment to facilitate stock control work, such as computers and computer programmes, among others. In terms of care activities, difficulties such as a lack of satisfactory knowledge about medicines, a lack of knowledge about legal dispensing rules and stronger relationships with other services and professionals outweighed the difficulties.

CHAPTER 5

FINAL CONSIDERATIONS

The concept of action is linked to the notion of freedom to act and transform the world which, for Heidegger, is not a place but a complex formed by the significance of the experiences that make the human being a historical being (MINAYO, 2012, p. 625).

This work does not end our reflections on the practice of dispensing medicines in the PSF; on the contrary, it shows the need for more in-depth reflection not only on dispensing itself, but on the whole process that the medicine goes through until it reaches its final destination, the user. However, we only analysed dispensing and its articulation in practice from the point of view of the different social actors involved in the work process.

Thus, based on this object of study, we synthesise our reflections under the aegis of our observations and the varied contributions of workers, managers and users on how the dispensing of medicines has been developed in the USF in a municipality in the semi-arid region of Bahia.

The organisation of the functioning of the SUS, created with the aim of establishing equal universal access to health service actions, including pharmacotherapy and pharmaceutical care, uses normative instruments such as the National Medicines Policy (PNM) and the National Pharmaceutical Care Policy (PNAF), which leads us to a perception of the complexity of regulating the pharmaceutical sector and the need to transform all this normative arsenal into health care, particularly in practices that promote the rational use of medicines.

In our study, managers attribute meanings and significance to pharmaceutical services that we were unable to confirm in our observations. For these informants, pharmaceutical services are a health policy, with defined stages and articulations that translate into real assistance for users. On the other hand, the non-pharmaceutical workers who took part in the study, who dispensed medicines, considered pharmaceutical services to be restricted to the mechanised act of handing over the medicine, carrying out physical checks and storing it in the pharmacy, and considered that this activity should be the pharmacist's duty.

Many difficulties were identified in the work process of dispensing medicines, since this is the responsibility of the nursing technician, but is routinely carried out by different actors, negating the manifestations of control, access and welcoming referenced by the nursing technicians. This situation leads us to the conclusion that there is no articulation between the actors responsible for user care, insofar as each one is limited to their training activity: doctors and dentists prescribe, nurses look after and manage the unit, technicians and others carry out the most varied activities under the supervision of the nurse.

In this scenario, personal relationships develop to a good standard, but there is no knowledge of each other's work or of their own care role, as communications do not involve the functions they fulfil or are not geared towards health care.

We also observed that the practice of dispensing is devoid of a humanised welcome, coupled with the proper handling of the medication that preserves its intrinsic qualities and favours its use with the aim of a therapy with positive results.

We therefore found that there are many difficulties and misunderstandings about working relationships, the structural conditions of pharmacies, the complete absence of pharmacists from primary care services, the distancing of central management from local problems, with a predominance of managerial actions to the detriment of care actions and particularly clinical pharmacy and pharmaceutical care.

The reality portrayed here is worrying, because dispensing practices lead to high health costs with medicines, which can lead to diversion and loss of medicines, inadequate disposal of expired medicines, dispensing mistakes and errors that can jeopardise users' lives. There are no pre-established procedures, as are required for the private sector of the medicines trade, there are no local protocols, nor compliance with those already recommended by the normative instruments of the Ministry of Health, included in the National Medicines Policy and the National Pharmaceutical Assistance Policy.

However, the managers are optimistic about the existing proposals at central level for expanding pharmaceutical assistance and implementing the municipal health plan, the advances in the sector such as the restructuring of the Pharmaceutical Supply Centre, better performance in the distribution of medicines with shorter supply times to the units, the creation of the Pharmacy and Therapeutics Commission, among other measures.

Even though we share the managers' optimism, our understanding leads us to a certain scepticism that quality, humanised access and the rational use of medicines can be achieved with one-off administrative actions. We recognise that the pharmaceutical care process is complex, but without any professional corporatism, the inclusion of pharmacists in the minimum PSF team and in the NASF is an indispensable starting point for implementing structural and conceptual changes in PS and particularly in the focus of our study to adopt dispensing practices and basic and indispensable criteria for the rational use of medicines.

On the other hand, user feedback is the first element to take into account in a project to restructure care. The level of discontent, disbelief and dissatisfaction among users corroborates our observations of a mechanised practice, centred on managerial activities and which does not guarantee universal access to medicines. The majority of users suffer from the precariousness of the units, ranging from the physical inadequacy of the pharmacies, the lack of medicines, the absence of professionals to give them proper guidance and the lack of a humanised welcome that pays attention to their basic needs, forcing them to migrate to hospital services in an attempt to have their demands met.

Therefore, based on the results of this study, we present some proposals that could contribute to changing the current situation regarding the dispensing of medicines in the family health units in the municipality of Feira de Santana. However, we would like to emphasise that the proposals and plans to be presented to the municipal health department are not simple tasks that can be carried out immediately, but rather point inexorably to the need for a starting point for change:

- An increase in the number of pharmacists, via competitive examination, as a way of eliminating turnover in the sector, both at central level and in the units with a larger catchment area.

- Creation of NASF teams with the inclusion of pharmacists in these teams;

- Training pharmacists in managerial activities, but especially in clinical pharmacy and pharmaceutical care.

- Creation of the Pharmacy and Therapeutics Commission at Central level and in the larger units, offering support to the other FH units;

- Adaptation of the physical spaces of the network's pharmacies in accordance with the Manual for the physical structure of basic health units: family health (BRASIL, 2006).

REFERENCES

ACURCIO, F. A. Medicines Policy and Pharmaceutical Assistance in the Unified Health System. In: ACURCIO, Francisco de Assis (Org.). **Medicamentos e Assistência Farmacêutica**. Belo Horizonte: Coopmed, 2003.

ALENCAR, T.O.S.; BASTOS, V.P.; ALENCAR, B. R.; FREITAS, I.V. Pharmaceutical dispensing: an analysis of legal concepts in relation to professional practice. **Revista de Ciências Farmacêuticas Básica e Aplicada,** v.32, n.1, p. 89-94, 2011.

ALENCAR, T.O.S.; NASCIMENTO, M.A.A.; ALENCAR, B. R. **Assistência farmacêutica no SUS:** articulating subjects, knowledge and practices. Feira de Santana UEFS Editora, 2011.

ALENCAR. B.R. Processo de Trabalho no Programa Saúde da Família: um enfoque na Assistência Farmacêutica. Dissertation presented to the Postgraduate Programme in Collective Health - Academic Master's Degree at the State University of Feira de Santana-UEFS. 2013

ALFOB. ASSOCIAÇÃO DOS LABORATÓRIOS FARMACÊUTICOS OFICIAIS DO BRASIL.

(ALFOB) Laboratórios Oficias do Brasil, 2012. Available at:<http://www.alfob.com.br>. Accessed on 30 Nov. 2012.

ANGONESI, D. Pharmaceutical dispensing: an analysis of different concepts and models. **Ciência &Saúde Coletiva,** v.13, p. 629-640, 2008.

ANGONESI, D.; RENNÓ, M.U.P. Pharmaceutical dispensing concepts and procedures: In **The Basics of Rational Drug Dispensing for Pharmacists.** São Paulo: Pharmabooks, 2012 p. 47

ANGONESI, D.; RENNÓ, M.U.P. Pharmaceutical dispensing: proposal of a model for practice. **Ciência & Saúde Coletiva,** v.16, n. 9, p. 3883-3891, 2011.

ARAÚJO, A.L.A.;PEREIRA, L.R.L.; UETA, J.M.; FREITAS, O. Assistência Farmacêutica como modelo tecnológico em atenção primária à saúde. **Revista de Ciências Farmacêuticas Básica e Aplicada.** V.26, n.2, p.87-92, 2005

ARAÚJO, A. L. A.; FREITAS, O. Conceptions of the pharmaceutical professional about pharmaceutical assistance in the basic health unit: difficulties and elements for change. **Revista Brasileira de Ciências Farmacêuticas,** v. 42, n. 1, p. 137-146, 2006.

ARAÚJO, A.L.A.;PEREIRA, L.R.L.; UETA, J.M.; FREITAS,O. Profile of pharmaceutical care in primary care of the Unified Health System. Ribeirão Preto, São Paulo **Ciência & Saúde Coletiva,** v.13 (Sup), p. 611-617, 2008.

ARAÚJO, A.L.A.;PEREIRA, L.R.L.; UETA, J.M.; FREITAS,O. Assistência Farmacêutica como um modelo tecnológico em atenção primária à saúde **Revista de Ciências Farmacêuticas Básicas Aplicadas** v.26, n.2, p. 611-617, 2008.

ARRAES, P.S.D.; BARRETO, M.L.; COELHO, H.L.L. Aspects of the processes of prescribing and dispensing medicines in the perception of the patient: a population-based study in Fortaleza, Ceará, Brazil. **Caderno de Saúde Pública.** v.23, n.4, p. 927-937, 2007.

ASSIS, M.M.A.; NASCIMENTO, M.A.A.; FRANCO, T.B.; JORGE,M.S.B. **Produção do cuidado no Programa Saúde da Família**: olhares analisadores em diferentes cenários. Salvador: EDUFBA, 2010.

ASSIS, M.M.A; JORGE, M.S.B. Methods of Analysis in Qualitative Research. In___ **Research.** Methods of understanding social reality. Feira de Santana: State University of Feira de Santana, 2010, p. 139-159.

BARBOSA D. M. **Atribuições do farmacêutico na atenção primária à saúde.** Dissertation presented to the Postgraduate Programme in Pharmaceutical Sciences at the Faculty of Pharmacy of the Federal University of Minas Gerais. 2009.

BARROS, D.M.; SÁ, M.C. O processo de trabalho em saúde e a produção do cuidado em uma unidade de saúde da família: limites ao acolhimento e reflexos no serviço de emergência. **Ciência & Saúde Coletiva,** v.15, n.5 p. 2473-2482, aug 2010

BARROS, J.A.C. **Propaganda de medicamentos-Atentados à Saúde?** São Paulo: Hucitec/Sobravime,

1995.

BERMUDEZ, J. Remédio: Saúde ou Indústria? The production of medicines in Brazil. Rio de Janeiro: Relume Dumará, 1992.

BEZZEGH,N.J; GOLDENBERG, P. The Challenge of Responsible dispensing: formal education versus professional practice.**Brasilian Journal of Pharmaceutical Sciences**, v.47,n.1,2011

BRAZIL **Law No. 5.991 of 17 December 1973.** Available at: <http://www.suvisa.rn.gov.br/contentproducao/aplicacao/suvisa/arquivos/gerados/lei_5.991_dezembro_1973.pdf>. Accessed on: 04 March 2013.

Ministry of Health. Medicines Centre. **1st National Meeting on Pharmaceutical Assistance and Medicines Policy**. Brasília-DF: Ministry of Health, 1988.

BRAZIL, National Health Council. **Resolution no. 196 of 10 October 1996.** Guidelines and regulatory standards for research involving humans. Brasília, DF: National Health Council, 1996.

BRAZIL, Ministry of Health. **Pharmaceutical Assistance in Primary Care:** technical instructions for its organisation. Brasília-DF Ministry of Health, 2002. p. 17-19.

BRAZIL, Ministry of Health. National Health Council. **Resolution No. 338, of 06 May 2004**, Approves the National Pharmaceutical Assistance Policy. Available at: <http://portal.saude.gov.br/portal/arquivos/pdf/reol_cns338.pdf. Accessed in Oct. 2011a>.

BRAZIL. FEDERAL COUNCIL OF PHARMACY. **Decree No. 85.878 of 07 April 1981.** The Legal Organisation of the Pharmaceutical Profession, 2000 p.343-344

BRAZIL, Ministry of Health. National Health Council. **Resolution No. 338, of 06 May 2004**, Approves the National Pharmaceutical Assistance Policy. Available at: <http://portal.saude.gov.br/portal/arquivos/pdf/reol_cns338.pdf>. Accessed in October 2011.

BRAZIL. Federal Pharmacy Council. **Resolution 499 of 17 December 2008.** Provides for the provision of pharmaceutical services in pharmacies and drugstores, and makes other provisions. Brasília-DF. Federal Pharmacy Council, 2008. Available at:< http://www.cff.org.br/userfiles/file/resolucoes/499.pdf >Accessed on: 15 September 2013.

BRAZIL. Federal Pharmacy Council. **Resolution n⁰ 357, of 20 April 2001.** Approves the technical regulation on Good Pharmacy Practices. Brasília-DF. Federal Pharmacy Council, 2001 Available at: <http://www.cff.org.br/userfiles/file/resoluções/357.pdf>. Accessed on: 18 de out.2011b.

BRAZIL. Federal Pharmacy Council. **Resolution 542 of 19 January 2011.** Provides for the duties of pharmacists in the dispensing and control of antimicrobials. Brasília-DF. Federal Pharmacy Council, 2011b. Available at: <http://www.cff.org.br/userfiles/file/resolucoes/542.pdf>. Accessed on: 23 March 2013.

BRAZIL. Federal Pharmacy Council. **Resolution No.** 585 **of 29 August 2013** Provides for the clinical attributions of pharmacists and makes other provisions.Brasília-DF. Federal Pharmacy Council,

2011c. Available at: <http://www.cff.org.br/userfiles/file/resolucoes/585.pdf>. Accessed on: 23 September 2013.

BRAZIL. Federal Pharmacy Council. **Resolution No. 586** of 29 August 2013 regulating pharmaceutical prescription and other measures.Brasília-DF. Federal Pharmacy Council, 2011c. Available at: <http://www.cff.org.br/userfiles/file/resolucoes/585.pdf>. Accessed on: 23 September 2013.

BRAZIL. Federal Pharmacy Council**. Resolution no. 308, of 2nd May 1997**. Provides for Pharmaceutical Assistance in pharmacies and drugstores. Brasília, DF: Federal Pharmacy Council, 1997. Available at:< http://www.cff.org.br/userfiles/file/resoluções/308.pdf>. Accessed on: 18 October 2011a.

BRAZIL. IBGE **Cities, 2012**. Feira de Santana. Available at <http://www.ibge.gov.br/cidadesat/xtras/perfil.php?codmun=291080#>. Accessed on: 15 March 2013.

BRAZIL. **Law n⁰ 8.080 of 19 September 1990**. Available at: <http://www.planalto.gov.br/ccivil_03/leis/8080htma>. Accessed on: 20 October 2012.

BRAZIL**. Law No. 9.782 of 26 January 1999** Defines the National Health Surveillance System, creates the National Health Surveillance Agency, and makes other provisions. Available at <http://portal.anvisa.gov.br/wps/content/Anvisa+Portal/Anvisa/Inicio/Laboratorios/>. Accessed on: 15 May 2013.

BRAZIL. Ministry of Health. **Ordinance No. 2488 of 21 October 2011**. Approves the National Primary Care Policy, establishing revised guidelines and norms for the organisation of Primary Care, the Family Health Strategy (ESF) and the Community Health Agents Programme (PACS). Brasília-DF: Ministry of Health, 2011d.
Available at <http://www.saúde.gov.br/dab>.. Accessed on 23 September 2013

BRAZIL. National Health Surveillance Agency. Resolution of the Collegiate Directorate-RDC no. 44, of 17 August 2009. Provides for Good Pharmaceutical Practices for the sanitary control of the operation, dispensing and commercialisation of products and the provision of pharmaceutical services in pharmacies and drugstores and makes other provisions. Brasília-DF: ANVISA, 2009. Available at <http://www.anvisa.gov.br>. Accessed on: 23 September 2013.

BRAZIL. Ministry of Health. Health Care Secretariat. Department of Primary Care. **National Primary Care Policy.** Brasília, DF: Ministry of Health 2006.

BRAZIL. Ministry of Health. Health Care Secretariat. Department of Primary Care**. Manual for the physical structure of basic family health units** Brasília, DF: Ministry of Health 2006.

BRAZIL. Ministry of Health NATIONAL HEALTH SURVEILLANCE AGENCY. **Terms of** Reference-National **Seminar** on Advertising and the Rational Use of Medicines. Brasilia, 2011a.

BRAZIL. Ministry of Health NATIONAL HEALTH COUNCIL, Resolution No. 466 of 12 December 2012 establishing the Guidelines and Regulatory Standards for Research Involving Human Beings <http://conselho.saude.gov.br/resolucoes/2012/Reso466.pdf> . Accessed on 20 September 2013.

BRAZIL. Ministry of Health. **Decree 7.508 of 28 July 2011** Regulates Law No·8.080 of 19 September 1990 to provide for the organisation of the Unified Health System (SUS), health planning, health care and inter-federative coordination, and makes other provisions. Brasília-DF: Ministry of Health, 2011c. Available at: <http://www.planalto.gov.br/ccivil_03/_ato2011-2014/2011/decreto/D7508.htm>. Accessed in Oct. 2013.

BRAZIL. Ministry of Health. **Ordinance No. 3.916 of 30 October 1998**. Approves the Medicines Policy. Brasília, DF: Ministry of Health, 1998. Available at: <http://www.saude.gov.br>. Accessed on: 12 December 2012.

CALADO, S.S. **Análise de documentos**: método de recolha e análise de dados. Master's Degree in Education - Didactics of Science University of Lisbon. 2005.

CARVALHO, M.C.R.D.; ACCIOLY JR,H.; RAFFIN,F.N.;CAMPOS, M.N.; CRUZ, M.M.C.; ALVES, M.K.S. Social representations of generic drugs by pharmacists: determination of central and peripheral systems. **Caderno de Saúde Pública.** v. 21 n. 1, p. 226-234, 2005

CARVALHO, L.J.M.A. Sobre a política de dispensação de medicamentos no Brasil: mínimo necessário para a efetivação do direito à saúde. **Revista Direito e Justiça-Reflexões** sociopolíticas. V.8, n.11, p. 159-169, 2010.

CASTRO, L. L. de; CALDAS, E. D. . Knowledge, practice and perception of the use of medicines in the Federal District. **Revista de Ciências Farmacêuticas Básica e Aplicada**, v. 32, p. 225-232, 2011.

CASTRO. L. L. C. de; COSTA, A. M. ; KOZOROSKI, A. ; ROSSINI, A. ; CYMROT, R. . Some Characteristics of the Practice of Self-Medication in Campo Grande, MS. **Revista de Ciências Farmacêuticas Básica e Aplicada**,v. 21, n.1, p. 81-101 2000.

CHAPELA, M. C.; SERAPIONI, M.; GASTALDO, D. Sobre el desencuentro salud colectiva: metodología cualitaiva. **Ciência & Saúde Coletiva**, vol.17, n.3, p. 587-594, 2012.

CIPOLLE, R. J.; STRAND, L.M.; MORLEY, P.C. **The Practice of Pharmaceutical Care.** Translation by Denise Borges Bittar. Brasília: Federal Pharmacy Council, p.396, 2006.

CORDEIRO, B. C.; LEITE, S.N. (Org.) **O Farmacêutico na atenção à Saúde.** Itajaí: UNIVALI Editora, p.79-81, 2008.

CORRER, C.J.; SOLER.O.; OTUKI,M.F. Assistência Farmacêutica integrada ao processo de cuidados em saúde: gestão clínica do medicamento. **Pan-Amazonian Health Journal**, v.2 p. 41-49, 2011

D'ÁVILA, L. S. **The work of dispensing medicines in a basic health unit in Belo Horizonte: a study of management and work activity.** Dissertation submitted to the Postgraduate Programme in Public Health at the Faculty of Medicine of the Federal University of Minas Gerais - UFMG, 2009.

DELLAMORA, E.C.L.; CAETANO, R.; CASTRO, C.G.S.O. Dispensing of medicines from the specialised component in centres in the state of Rio de Janeiro. **Ciência & Saúde Coletiva,** v. 17 p. 2387-2396, 2012.

FEIRA DE SANTANA. Municipal Health Department. Primary Care Department. **Primary Care Management Report.** Feira de Santana-BA 2013.

FONTANELLA, B.J.B.; LUCHESI, B.M; SAIDEL, M.G.B; B.J.B; RICAS, J ; TURATO, E.R; MELO, D.G. Sampling in qualitative research: proposal of procedures to verify theoretical saturation.**Ciência & Saúde Coletiva** v. 27, n. 2 p.389-394, feb. 2011.

FONTANELLA,. Saturation sampling in qualitative health research: theoretical contributions. **Caderno de Saúde Pública**, v.24, n.2 p.17, jan, 2008

G, C. A. P. **"Pharmaceutical Assistance in Brazil: Analysis and Perspectives."** *Secretary of Health Policies. Ministry of Health, Brasília-DF* (2012).

GOMES JR, E. A. **Prevalence of the use of medicines without medical prescription by users of the Basic Health Unit of the Cidade Nova neighbourhood, Feira de Santana-BA.**
Monograph on a course conclusion defended at the State University of Feira de Santana. 2009.

GOMES R. R.F. M; MACHADO C. J; ACURCIO,F.A; GUIMARÃES ,D.C. Use of pharmacy dispensing records as an indicator of non-adherence to antiretroviral therapy in HIV-infected individuals. **Caderno de . Saúde Pública**, Rio de Janeiro,v. 25,n.3, p.495-506, 2009.

GALATO, D., ALANO, G. M., TRAUTHMAN, S. C., & VIEIRA, A. C. (2008). Dispensing medicines: a reflection on the process for preventing, identifying and resolving problems related to pharmacotherapy.**Revista BrasileiraCiências Farmacêuticas**, v.44, n.3 jul/set, p.466-475.2008.

IBGE Cidades.< http://cidades.ibge.gov.br/xtras/perfil.php?codmun=291080> Accessed Oct. 2013.

IVAMA, A.M. *et.al.* Pharmaceutical Care in Brazil: "Treading Paths" Workshop Report. Brasília-DF: Pan American Health Organisation, 2001. p. 43

JESUS, E. B. Human Knowledge: challenges, adventure, risks, achievements... a continuous learning process. In___Research**.** Methods of understanding social reality. Feira de Santana: Universidade Estadual de Feira de Santana, 2010 p. 15-33.

LAKATOS, E. M; MARCONI, M. A. **Técnicas de pesquisa:** planejamento e execução de pesquisas; amostragem e técnicas de pesquisa; elaboração e interpretação de dados**.** 3.ed. São Paulo: Atlas, 1996.

LAVILLE, C.; DIONNE, J. **The construction of knowledge: a** manual of research methodology in the humanities. Porto Alegre. Ed. UFMG/ArtMED, 1999.

LEITE, S.N.; CORDEIRO, B.C. **O Farmacêutico na atenção à saúde**. Itajaí; Univale editora, 2008 p. 64-65.

LYRA JR., MARQUES, T.C.(Org.) Social Determination of the Health-Disease Process: the symbolic value of medicines and the medicalisation of society In:______ **The Bases of Rational Dispensing of Medicines for Pharmacists.** São Paulo: Pharmabooks, 2012 p. 9

LYRA JR., MESQUITA, A.R. Communication skills as a tool for the relationship between the pharmacist and the user In: ________________ , **As Bases da Dispensação Racional de Medicines for Pharmacists.** São Paulo: Pharmabooks, 2012 p. 99

MAGALHÃES, J.L; ANTUNES, A.M.S; BOECHT,N. Official pharmaceutical laboratories and their relevance to public health in Brazil. **RECIIS - R. Eletr. de Com. Inf. Inov. Saúde.** Rio de Janeiro, v5, n.1, p.85-99, Mar., 2011

MARIN, N. (Org). **Pharmaceutical Assistance for Municipal Managers.** Rio de Janeiro: Pan American Health Organisation/World Health Organisation, 2003.

MARX, K. **Capital.** 14 ed. Rio de Janeiro. Bertrand Brasil 1994.

MENDES-GONÇALVES, R.B. **Práticas de saúde:** processo de trabalho e necessidades. São Paulo CEFOR 1992. 53p. Cadernos CEFOR. p.15.

MENDES-GONÇALVES, R.B. **Tecnologia e Organização Social das práticas de saúde.** São Paulo: Hucitec-Abrasco 1994 p. 126

MENEZES, T.M.O; GUIMARÃES,E.P; SANTOS, E.M.P; NASCIMENTO,M.V;ARAUJO,P.D .G rupo educativo com dispensação de medicamentos: uma estratégiaade adesão ao tratamento da hipertensão arterial e do diabetes mellitus.Revista Baiana de Saúde Pública, v.36, n.1, p148-158, 2012

MERHY, E.E In search of quality in health services: open door health services and the techno-healthcare model in defence of life. in: Luiz Carlos de Oliveira (org.) **Inventing Change in Health.** São Paulo: HUCITEC, 1994, P. 117-160

MERHY, E.E.;ONOCKO.R. **Acting in Health.** A challenge for the public. 2 ed. São Paulo: Hucitec 2006.

MINAYO, M.C.S. Qualitative analysis: theory, steps and reliability. **Ciência & Saúde Coletiva,** vol.17, n.3, p. 621-626, 2012.

MINAYO, M.C.S. **Desafio do conhecimento: pesquisa qualitativa em saúde.** 12 ed. São Paulo. Hucitec/ABRASCO, 2010.

MINAYO, M.C.S. **Desafio do conhecimento:** pesquisa qualitativa em saúde. 8. ed. São Paulo. Hucitec/ABRASCO, 2004.

MOTA.D.M.et al. Rational use of medicines: an economic approach for decision-making. **Ciência & Saúde Coletiva,** v.13, p. 589 - 601,2008.

NASCIMENTO, A. Is this regulation? 1st edition, São Paulo. Sobravime, 2005

OENNING,D.;OLIVEIRA, B.V; BLATT, C.R. Patients' knowledge of prescribed medicines after medical consultation and dispensation. **Ciência & Saúde Coletiva,** v.16, n. 7, p. 3277-3273, 2011.

WORLD HEALTH ORGANISATION. Rational use of medicines. **Report of the Conference of**

Experts. Nairobi, 25-29 November 1993 Geneva.

PERINI, E. Pharmaceutical Services: theoretical and conceptual foundations. In: Francisco de Assis Acurcio.(org.) **Medicamentos e Assistência Farmacêutica**. Belo Horizonte: Coopmed Editora Médica, 2003.

PIOVISCHINI, A. R. **Pé de mim**. In: Arcos de Mercúrio - Anthologia Poética do Tarô / Enrique Sampaio, Larissa Rodrigues, Will Fialho, organisation and sealing. Feira de Santana: Diabo A4 Ed., 2015. Pag. 37.

RAMOS. D, SILVA. T.O.; ALENCAR. B.R. Análise da prática do estoque domiciliar de edicamentos em um município do Estado da Bahia. **Infarma,** v.22. n. 9-10, p. 50-5, 2010.

ROCHA, S.M.M.,ALMEIDA,M.C. P. O processo de trabalho da enfermagem em saúde coletiva e a interdisciplinaridade. **Latin American Journal of Nursing.** Rio de Janeiro v.8 n.6, Dec 2000.

ROZENFELD, S. Pharmacist: health professional and citizen. **Ciência & Saúde Coletiva**. v.13 (suppl). Rio de Janeiro. apr. 2008.

SANTANA, J.S.S. Methodological Path. In: SANTANA, J.S.S; NASCIMENTO, M.A.A (ORG.) **Pesquisa.** Methods of understanding social reality. Feira de Santana: State University of Feira de Santana, 2010, p. 87-119.

SANTOS.V, NITRINI. S.M.O.O, Indicators of prescription drug use and patient care in health services. **Revista de Saúde Pública.** n. 38, v.6, p. 819-26. 2004

SANTOS, A. C. Desenvolvimento, Civilização e Modernidade:O sonho da industrialização em Feira de Santana.< http://www.klepsidra.net/klepsidra15/feira.htm>. Accessed Oct. 2013

SEVALHO, G. Medicines perceived as hybrid objects: a critical view of rational use. **In: ACURCIO, F. A. (Org.) Medicamentos e Assistência Farmacêutica**. Belo Horizonte. Coopmed, 2003.

SOARES, S.L.; DIEHL, E.E.; LEITE, S.N.;FARIAS, M. R. A Model for drug dispensing service based on the care process in the Brazilian Helth System. **Brazilian Journal of Pharmaceutical Sciences**. V.49, n.1 jan/mar., 2013

VALLADÃO,M.L.F; LISBOA,S.M; FERNANDES, C. Prescriptions and pharmaceutical dispensing; a health issue. **Revista Médica Minas Gerais,** v.14,p.21-25, 2004

VELLOSO, V.P. **Assistência Farmacêutica.** Discourse and practices in the capital of the Brazilian empire (1850-1880), Belo Horizonte: Varia História v.26, n.44, p.37.

VIEIRA, F.S.; MENDES, A.C.R. Evolution of the Ministry of Health's Spending on Medicines. Brasília: Ministry of Health, 2009. Available at: <http://portal.saude.gov.br/portal/arquivos/pdf/estudo_gasto_medicamentos.pdf>. Accessed on: 10 October 2012.

ZANINE, A.C.; OGA, S. Rational use of medicines. In: _______ **Applied Pharmacology**. 5.ed. São Paulo. Atheneu, 1994. p.684-691.

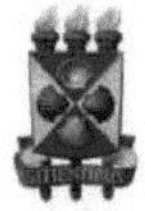

APPENDIX A
State University of Feira de Santana
Health Department
Postgraduate Programme in Collective Health
Master's in Collective Health

Research title: Medicines Dispensing Practices in Family Units
Researcher: Inalva Valadares Freitas
Supervisor: Prof[1]. DP Maria Angela A. do Nascimento

SYSTEMATIC OBSERVATION SCRIPT

Observation of the practice of dispensing medicines:

- Structure of the pharmacy in the family health unit;
- Initial reception and dialogue with the user;
- Organisation of the service;
- Storage of medicines;
- Dispensing itself:
    - Prescription evaluation process
    - Use of lightweight technology;
    - Use of light-hard and hard technology.

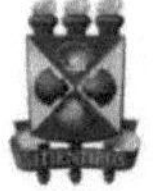

APPENDIX B
State University of Feira de Santana
Health Department
Postgraduate Programme in Collective Health
Master's in Collective Health

Research title: Medicines Dispensing Practices in Family Units in a municipality in the state of Bahia
Researcher: Inalva Valadares Freitas
Supervisor: ProP. DP Maria Angela A. do Nascimento

SEMI-STRUCTURED INTERVIEW SCRIPT
(Pharmacists and other workers directly involved in dispensing)

DATE: ____/ ____/ ____
Entry no:
Inicio:
End:

1) Characterisation of the interviewee:

a) Sex:

b) Age:
c) Year of completion of training course (undergraduate or technical)
d) Length of professional experience in **primary** care:

2) Guiding themes:

2.1 Work process in the practice of dispensing medicines
- concept of dispensation;
- subject of the labour process;
- object of work;
- activities carried out;
- instruments used for dispensing medicines.

2.2 Interpersonal relations between workers/users
- reception
- bond
- resolvability
- access

2.3 Difficulties/facilities encountered in carrying out dispensing activities.

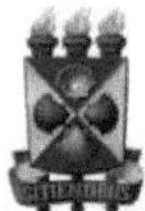

APPENDIX C
State University of Feira de Santana
Health Department
Postgraduate Programme in Collective Health
Master's in Collective Health

Research title: Medicines Dispensing Practices in Family Units in a municipality in the state of Bahia
Researcher: Inalva Valadares Freitas
Supervisor: ProP. DP Maria Angela A. do Nascimento

SEMI-STRUCTURED INTERVIEW SCRIPT
(Users)

DATE: ____/ ____/ ____
Entry no:
Inicio:
End:

2) Characterisation of the interviewee:

a) Sex:
b) Age:
c) Education
d) Profession/occupation

3) Guiding themes:

3.1 Interpersonal relations between workers/users
- reception
- bond
- resolvability
- access

- Dispensing activities ;

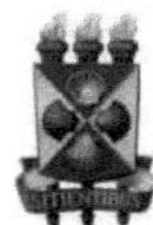

APPENDIX D

State University of Feira de Santana

Health Department
Postgraduate Programme in Collective Health
Master's in Collective Health

Research title: Medicines Dispensing Practices in Family Units in a municipality in the state of Bahia
Researcher: Inalva Valadares Freitas
Supervisor: Prof[1]. DP Maria Angela A. do Nascimento

SEMI-STRUCTURED INTERVIEW SCRIPT

(Managers)

DATE: ____/ ____/ ____
Entry no:
Inicio:
End:

3 Characterisation of the interviewee:

a) Sex:
b) Age:
c) Year of graduation:
d) Length of professional experience

2 Guiding themes:

2.1 Understanding the practice of dispensing medicines;
2.2 Work process in the practice of dispensing medicines;
2.3 Liaising with other professionals in the Unit;
2.4 Difficulties/facilities in dispensing medicines;

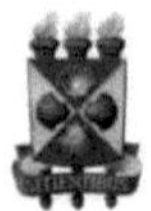

APPENDIX E
Informed Consent Form

I, Inalva Valadares Freitas, the researcher in charge, and collaborating researcher Professor Maria Angela Alves do Nascimento from the Centre for Integrated Research in Collective Health (NUPISC) at the State University of Feira de Santana (UEFS), invite you to take part in a study on the practice of dispensing medicines in pharmacies in family health units, with the aim of analysing this practice of dispensing medicines. This study could contribute to the adoption of strategies and policies that help the pharmaceutical profession, and thus improve users' access to medicines, as well as promoting their correct and beneficial use. In order to collect the data, it will be necessary to interview you and observe the dispensing service. If you take part in the research, you will not incur any financial costs, you will not be identified, and you will have a private place to be interviewed, free from listening to and observing other people. You will be guaranteed secrecy and confidentiality during and after the interviews, which will be recorded if you allow it. The tapes and observations will be kept for five years at the Centre for Integrated Research in Collective Health (NUPISC), under our care, after which time they will be destroyed. We will take every care to respect your physical, psychological, moral, intellectual, social, cultural and spiritual integrity, in the event of any immediate or delayed damage, in order to avoid any harmful consequences with regard to the free expression of your opinions. We would like to point out that the possible risks of this research may be related to you feeling embarrassed, afraid or uncomfortable about answering any questions, but you can withdraw at any time from taking part in the study, or not answer the question. If the researchers notice any damage or risk to your health during the course of the research, it will be stopped immediately and we will give you all the necessary attention. Regarding the results of the research, they will be forwarded and presented to the family health units you attend and you will be informed of the results. Please note that at any time you can ask the researchers for clarification about the research, who can be reached Monday to Friday at the UEFS Postgraduate Centre in Collective Health - Module 6-NUPISC Av. Transnordestina S/N Campus Universitário de Feira de Santana, telephone number (75) 3161-8162. Please note that the research will only be presented at scientific events such as congresses, symposiums, seminars and published in periodicals, scientific journals, books, among others. Once you have been informed about the research, if you agree to take part, you must sign this consent form in duplicate with the researchers, keeping a copy of it.
Feira de Santana, ____of__________________2013

____
Interviewee

__________________________ __________________________
Inalva Valadares Freitas Maria Angela Alves do Nascimento

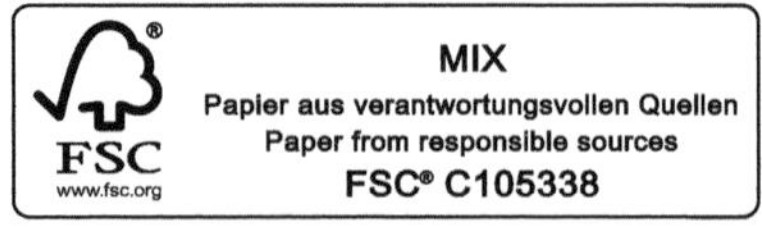

Printed by Books on Demand GmbH, Norderstedt / Germany